Handbook of Synthetic Substrates

HANDBOOK OF SYNTHETIC SUBSTRATES

For the Coagulation and Fibrinolytic System

by

H.C. HEMKER

Department of Biochemistry
Faculty of Medicine
University of Limburg
Maastricht, The Netherlands

with contributions by
M.C.E. VAN DAM-MIERAS
S. IWANAGA
C.M. JACKSON
J.M. NIGRETTO
K.C. ROBBINS

1983 **MARTINUS NIJHOFF PUBLISHERS**
a member of the KLUWER ACADEMIC PUBLISHERS GROUP
BOSTON / THE HAGUE / DORDRECHT / LANCASTER

Distributors

for the United States and Canada: Kluwer Boston, Inc., 190 Old Derby Street, Hingham, MA 02043, USA
for all other countries: Kluwer Academic Publishers Group, Distribution Center, P.O.Box 322, 3300 AH Dordrecht, The Netherlands

Library of Congress Cataloging in Publication Data   CIP

Hemker, H. C.
   Handbook of synthetic substrates for the coagulation
and fibrinolytic system.

   Bibliography: p.
   Includes index.
   1. Blood--Coagulation. 2. Fibrinolysis. 3. Chromo-
genic compounds--Analysis. I. Dam-Mieras, M. C. E. van.
II. Title.
QP93.5.H44 1983   612'.115   82-24678
ISBN-13:978-94-009-6692-5   e-ISBN-13:978-94-009-6690-1
DOI: 10.1007/978-94-009-6690-1   87-28241

ISBN-13:978-94-009-6692-5

Copyright

Contents

Preface   IX

Foreword   XI

I. Basic enzymology   1

I. 1.   Introduction   1
I. 2.   Maximal velocity   3
I. 3.   Michaelis constant   4
I. 4.   Low substrate concentration;
        the efficiency of an enzyme   5
I. 5.   High substrate concentration;
        the saturation curve   6
I. 6.   The characteristic parameters of an enzymatic
        reaction   7
I. 7.   Enzyme inhibition   9
I. 8.   Rate-constants and enzymatic mechanism   10
I. 9.   The reaction mechanism of serine proteases   12
I.10.   Transient state kinetics   16
I.11.   Data from a reaction going to completion   17
I.12.   Active site titration   18
I.13.   Simultaneous reactions in complicated reaction
        mixtures   21

II. Measuring the conversion of a chromogenic substrate   27

II. 1.   Photometric assays   27
II. 2.   Absorption spectrophotometry   28
II. 3.   Choice of wavelength and absorbancy range   32
II. 4.   Temperature   33
II. 5.   The reaction medium   35

II. 6.   Substrate solution   36
II. 7.   Methodology   38
II. 8.   Execution of the experiment   38
II. 9.   Fluorescence   44
II.10.   Electrochemical determinations   47

III. Substrates   53

III.1.   Specificity in serine proteases   53
III.2.   Substrate selectivity and sensitivity   57
III.3.   Inhibition by artificial substrates   64
III.4.   Data on commercially available substrates   65
III.5.   Fluorogenic substrates   83
III.6.   General principles of fluorogenic peptide substrates
          with 7-amino-4-methylcoumarine (MCA) as a leaving
          group   83
III.7.   Thioesters   88
III.8.   Substrates for electrochemical determinations   89
III.9.   Luminogenic substrates   90

IV. Determinations that can be carried out with chromogenic
     substrates   95

IV.1.   Thrombin and derived determinations   95
   1.1. thrombin   96
   1.2. prothrombin   96
   1.3. antithrombin III and heparin cofactor   98
   1.4. prothrombinase, factor V, platelet factor 3   99
   1.4.1. prothrombinase   100
   1.4.2. factor V   101
   1.4.3. platelet factor 3   101

IV.2.   Factor X_a and derived determinations   102
   2.1. factor X_a 102
   2.2. factor X   103
   2.3. antifactor X_a (antithrombin III,
         heparin cofactor)   104
   2.4. heparin   105
   2.5. platelet factor 4 and other antiheparins   106
   2.6. factor X activating enzymes   107

2.6.1. factor VIII   108
2.6.2. factor IX   108
2.6.3. platelet factor 3   108
2.6.4. factor VII and tissue thromboplastin   108

IV.3.   Determination of fibrinolytic pathway components
        in plasma   109
   3.1. plasminogen   109
   3.2. plasminogen activator   110
   3.3. 'free' protease activity   110
   3.4. plasmin generation rates   111
   3.5. α_2-plasmin inhibitor   111

IV.4.   The contact activation system   112
   4.1. plasma prekallikrein   112
   4.2. factor XII   114
   4.3. activated factor XI   116

IV.5.   Miscellaneous determinations   117
   5.1. glandular kallikrein   117
   5.2. brinase and brinase inhibitors   118
   5.3. bacterial endotoxins   119

Bibliography of synthetic substrates (as available Fall 1982)   125

Index of subjects   169

Preface

The need for a handbook on the use of synthetic substrates for assay of proteases of the coagulation and fibrinolytic systems became evident several years ago during the activities of the Subcommittee on Synthetic Substrates of the International Committee on Thrombosis and Haemostasis (ICTH). Production of such a handbook, which was recommended during discussions of the ICTH at its meeting in London in 1979 was made possible by the generous efforts of Professor HC Hemker with the aid of several contributors with particular interests in the use of synthetic substrates in coagulation and fibrinolysis. As current Chairman and Secretary General of the ICTH we would like to express our sincere thanks to Professor Hemker for producing this handbook and look forward to seeing the benefits of this tremendous effort reflected in the advancement of our understanding of thrombosis and hemostasis and the transfer of such knowledge into improved diagnosis and treatment of thrombotic and hemorrhagic disorders.

Craig M Jackson
Professor of Biological Chemistry
Washington University School of Medicine, St. Louis, MO
Chairman, ICTH

Harold R Roberts
Professor of Internal Medicine
University of North Carolina, Chapel Hill, NC
Secretary General, ICTH

Foreword

The advent of synthetic substrates for the study of bloodcoagulation and fibrinolysis was a significant step forward in the investigation of these systems. Both basic research and clinical laboratory investigations can profit from these advanced tools.

The International Committee on Thrombosis and Haemostasis, through its subcommittee on chromogenic substrates, rapidly became aware that the progress possible in this field could be improved by the presentation in a concise form of the relevant information available.

The necessary information appeared to come in four kinds:

1) *Basic knowledge on enzyme kinetics.*
   This is mandatory for understanding the use of chromogenic substrates, but it is not standard knowledge of the coagulation pathophysiologist.
2) *The scientific basis of the practise of the measuring techniques.*
   This contains the necessary background information for the new types of benchwork introduced in the coagulation laboratory.
3) *The product information,* including the enzyme kinetic data of the various substrates. As yet these were available in many scattered publications only.
4) *An overview of the coagulation and fibrinolysis methods in which synthetic substrates have been employed.*

These four kinds of information are given in the four chapters of this book. A substantial part of the contents of this book is based on paragraphs contributed by scientists known to be experts in different aspects of the use of synthetic substrates. These paragraphs, listed below in alphabetical order, were especially written for this book.

1) S Iwanaga, H Kato, T Morita, T Sugo, Y Ohno, M Ohki, K. Takada, S Sakakibara (Faculty of Sciences, Kyushu University, Fukuoka, Japan),
   Fluorogenic substrate assay methods for proteinases in blood coagulation, kallikrein-kinin and fibrinolysis systems.
2) CM Jackson (Washington University School of Medicine, St Louis, MO, U.S.A.),

Methods for increasing the specificity of chromogenic and fluorogenic substrate assays of plasma proteases.

3) JM Nigretto, M Jozefowicz (Université de Paris Nord, Villetaneuse, France),

Electrochemical activity determination of trypsin-like enzymes in whole blood using electrogenic substrates.

4) KC Robbins, RC Wohl (Michael Reese Research Foundation, Chicago, Ill, U.S.A.),

Determination of fibrinolytic pathway components in plasma.

I edited these contributions in order to obtain a certain unification of presentation and to prevent duplications. Except for these minor adaptations the manuscripts have been incorporated in the text unaltered.

A first draft of the text was circulated among the thirty main researchers active in the field of synthetic substrates. I would like to thank them for their suggestions, corrections and remarks, all of which have had their impact on the final version.

For reasons beyond my control the preparation of the final version has taken much more time than foreseen. Dr van Dam-Mieras (Department of Biochemistry, Faculty of Medicine, University of Limburg, Maastricht) has rewritten some parts of the text, contributed other parts and has seen to it that the references have been kept up to date. The Bibliography added at the end of the book also has been prepared by her.

I hope that the book will serve its purpose.

HC Hemker

Maastricht, Spring 1983

I. Basic enzymology

Summary

In the first paragraphs of this chapter (1−6) it is attempted to give an explanation of enzyme kinetics in such a form that those without previous knowledge of this matter can use it as an introduction. Basic information of this kind is necessary for the understanding of the use and applications of chromogenic substrates.

The further paragraphs are not compulsory reading for the understanding of the rest of the chapters but treat subjects that may become important under circumstances. Enzyme inhibition is treated in paragraph 7 a.o. because unwanted inhibition by competition between artificial and natural substrates can cause confusion in practise.

Paragraphs 8, 9 and 10 link the formalism of kinetics with the chemical events taking place in the reaction medium. Paragraph 11 discusses the information that can be obtained from a reaction going to completion. Active site titration, which is the cornerstone of standardisation in this field is discussed in paragraph 12 whereas the subject of simultaneous reactions, as they often occur in plasma, is treated in the last paragraph.

I.1. Introduction

An enzyme is a protein that due to its specific action can convert molecules, called the substrate(s) into others, called the product(s). As all catalysts an enzyme accelerates a reaction without being converted itself and without influencing the chemical equilibrium. This text concerns the assessment of the *enzymes* active in blood coagulation and fibrinolysis. We, therefore, will need a discussion of the basic concepts in enzymology. Blood coagulation and fibrinolysis factors are examples of those (pro)enzymes known as the serine proteases, therefore, we will treat general enzymology only insofar as it pertains to that class of enzymes. Also we cover the theory of enzyme action only insofar as it is necessary for the practice of using chromogenic substrates. For a

1

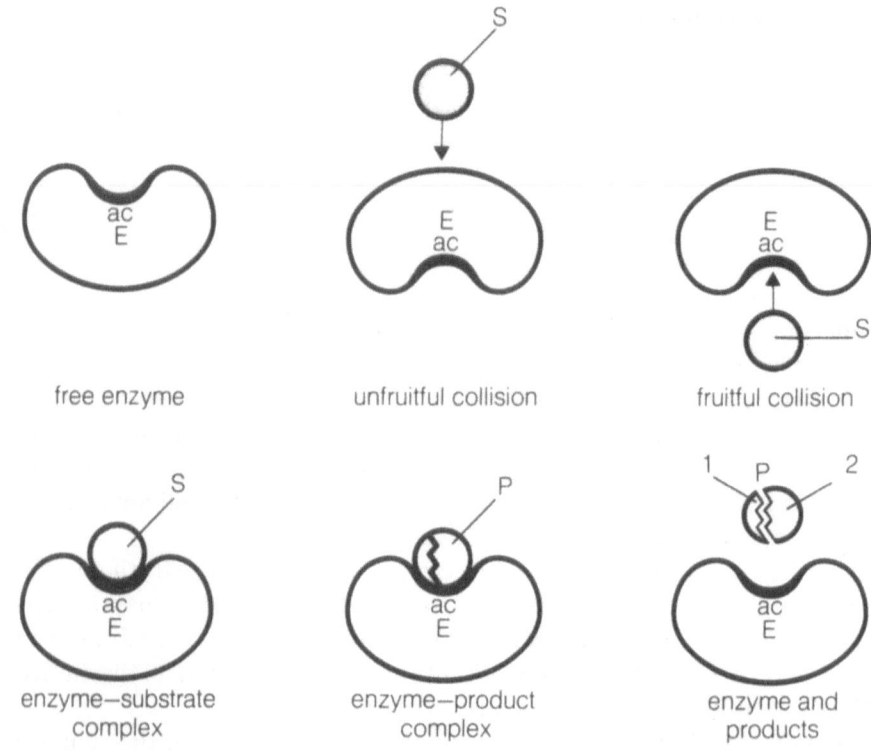

Fig. I.1. Time lapse 'photograph' of an enzymatic reaction. E = enzyme; S = substrate; ac = active centre; P = product.

more general treatment, the reader is explicitly referred to texts on enzymology (1–10).

Proteolytic enzymes are able to split amide bonds in proteins and peptides as well as ester bonds in certain esters. They act on one substrate at the time (not counting the water molecule involved in the lysis) and make two products in splitting it. They are often relatively nonspecific, that is they accept a broader spectrum of different substrates than most other enzymes do. If one tries to imagine what an enzyme molecule (E) does when it is active in a solution, one may get the following picture (Fig. I.1): the enzyme molecule from time to time collides with a substrate molecule (S). This collision may or may not lead to the formation of the so-called enzyme substrate complex (ES). If an enzyme substrate complex results we will speak of a 'fruitful' collision. In this complex the substrate is bound to the enzyme by a combination of weak interactions not involving covalent chemical bonds. The complex may fall apart into its constituent entities, or it may, by an intramolecular rearrangement of covalent bonds, convert into an enzyme-product complex. The latter complex then dissociates into the product and unchanged enzyme. In chemical formula $E + S \rightleftharpoons ES \rightarrow E + P$. The portion of the enzyme molecule directly involved in the chemical conversion, i.e. the residues that form and break covalent bonds, is called the *active site* of the enzyme.

One single enzyme molecule in the presence of its substrate will be either connected with a substrate molecule (ES) or free (E). The activity of such an enzyme molecule will be determined by the number of collisions that lead to enzyme-substrate complex formation and the rate at which a complex dissociates into enzyme and product. The time course of the events encountered by such an enzyme molecule can be depicted in the following way:

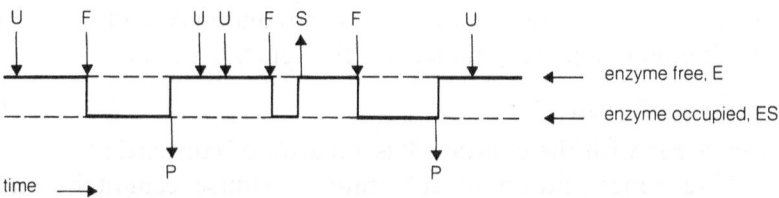

Fig. I.2. Life-line of an enzyme molecule. In this diagram the enzyme is shown to be alternatively in the free and occupied state. A fruitful collision leads to the occupied state which ends by the formation of free enzyme and product or falls apart in free enzyme and substrate. U = unfruitful collision; F = fruitful collision; P = product formation; S = substrate leaving the complex.

Both the collision frequencies and the life-time of the complex will vary statistically, but average values can be conveniently used. The fact that an increase in temperature will increase the reaction velocity can be easily understood from this model. At higher temperatures the number of collisions between substrate and enzyme will be higher, also the covalent bonds are less stable and will break earlier. Therefore, P will be more readily formed.

I.2. Maximal velocity, $V_{\max}$

We cannot imagine what an infinitely large substrate concentration would mean. Yet it is a convenient abstraction often used in enzymology. Infinite substrate concentration means a maximal number of fruitful collisions. So under these conditions each enzyme molecule will occur in the occupied form only (Fig. I.3).

The rate of product formation will be determined by the lifetime of the enzyme-substrate complex and by the number of complexes that

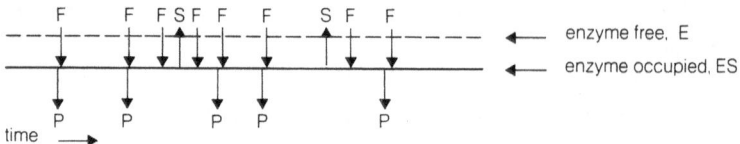

Fig. I.3. Life-line of an enzyme at infinite substrate concentration. (Meaning of the letters as in Fig. 2.). Each product formation is immediately followed by a fruitful collision.

are converted into enzyme-product complexes and thereafter dissociate forming a product. When the reaction conditions (temperature, pH etc.) are fixed, the number of fruitful collisions and the mean lifetime of complexes will be constant. So under saturating conditions each enzyme molecule will produce a product at a constant and maximally high speed. In a solution containing many molecules the velocity will be

$$V_{max} = k_{cat} \cdot E \qquad (1.1)$$

The subscript *cat* with the constant k is a matter of convention.

An infinite concentration of substrate of course cannot be realized in practice, but V_{max} can be calculated from velocities at known concentrations. V_{max} at unit enzyme concentration equals k_{cat}. This is an important constant in enzyme kinetics. It has the dimension of $time^{-1}$. It reflects the amount of substrate molecules one molecule of enzyme can handle per unit time, also called the *turnover number*. Values of k_{cat} for a proteolytic enzyme have a broad range between 10^{-2} and 10^{+8} turnovers per second; depending on the nature of both the enzyme and the substrate.

I.3. Michaelis constant K_m

The constant k_{cat} effectively quantitates what happens when the enzyme is completely occupied with substrate. In all realistic situations, however, there are finite concentrations of substrate present and therefore the enzyme will not be completely occupied. The reaction velocity in that case will be lower than the maximal velocity and proportional to the number of enzyme molecules that is occupied out of the total number or (which is the same) to the fraction of all the enzyme molecules that are occupied. The higher the substrate concentration, the higher the enzyme occupation.

Now there are unfruitful collisions, that do not lead to the formation of a complex. There are unfruitful dissociations of the complex as well, that do not yield a product but simply give back enzyme and substrate.

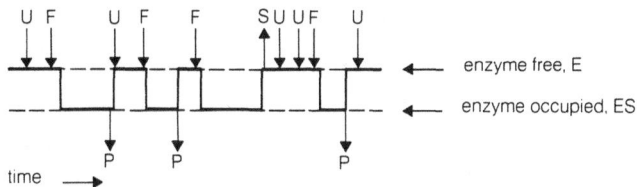

Fig. I.4. Life-line of an enzyme when the substrate concentration equals the Michaelis constant. Meaning of the letters as in Fig. I.2. At $S = K_m$ the enzyme is half occupied and the reaction velocity consequentially is half maximal.

How many of the encounters between enzyme and substrate lead to product formation depends on the characteristics of each enzyme-substrate pair. Different species of substrate will lead to different degrees of occupation of the enzyme at the same substrate concentrations. In order to quantitate this effect one can estimate the concentration of substrate that will lead to half occupation of the enzyme and hence to half maximal reaction velocity. This concentration is called K_m or Michaelis constant. K_m and k_{cat} together describe in a quantitative way the dependence of reaction velocity upon enzyme and substrate concentration.

I.4. Low substrate concentrations, the efficiency of an enzyme

At low substrate concentration the great majority of enzyme molecules will be unoccupied. The collisions between enzyme and substrate therefore will mostly be between the substrate and the unoccupied enzyme. Therefore, the number of collisions will be roughly proportional to the amount of substrate present. A certain number of the collisions will lead to a productive enzyme substrate complex i.e. an enzyme substrate complex that does yield a product. The higher the number of productive collisions, the more efficient the enzyme acts. This can be quantitated in an 'efficiency constant'. It stands to reason that the efficiency constant is proportional to k_{cat}, the catalytic constant discussed in paragraph I.2.

It also is easily seen intuitively that an enzyme is less efficient when it needs a higher concentration of substrate to obtain its half maximal reaction velocity. The efficiency constant thus can be felt to be inversely proportional to K_m. In the next paragraph we will see these relationships as part of a unifying formula, now we arrive intuitively at the following formula for reaction velocities at low substrate concentrations:

$$V = \frac{k_{cat}}{K_m} E.S. \tag{1.2}$$

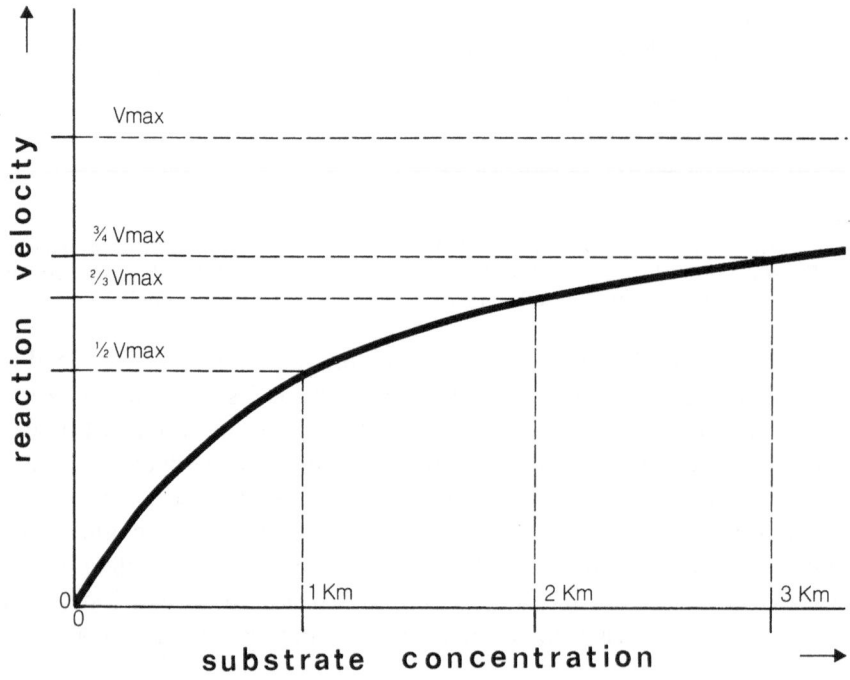

Fig. I.5. Graphic representation of reaction velocity (v) as a function of substrate concentration (S). At K_m the reaction velocity is half maximal. Only at an infinite substrate concentration the reaction velocity reaches V_{max}.

where the magnitude of k_{cat}/K_m is an indication of the efficiency of the enzyme. Here and in following formulas E and S stand for the Molar concentrations of Enzyme and Substrate resp.

I.5. High substrate concentration, the saturation curve

At higher substrate concentrations it will be increasingly difficult for substrate molecules to find an enzyme molecule that is not already occupied. At $S = K_m$ half of the enzyme molecules is occupied (or each molecule is occupied for half of the time). When the substrate concentration is twice K_m, $\frac{2}{3}$ of the enzyme will be occupied. In general when the substrate concentration is n times K_m, a fraction of $n/(n + 1)$ of the enzyme will be occupied, and the reaction velocity will be $n/(n + 1)$ times V_{max}. For n (and therefore S) approaching infinity, the enzyme will be saturated with substrate and v will approach V_{max}. This is illustrated in Fig. I.5. The velocity will always remain directly proportional to the amount of enzyme added. By its action the enzyme will bring about a decrease of substrate concentration and therefore of the velocity

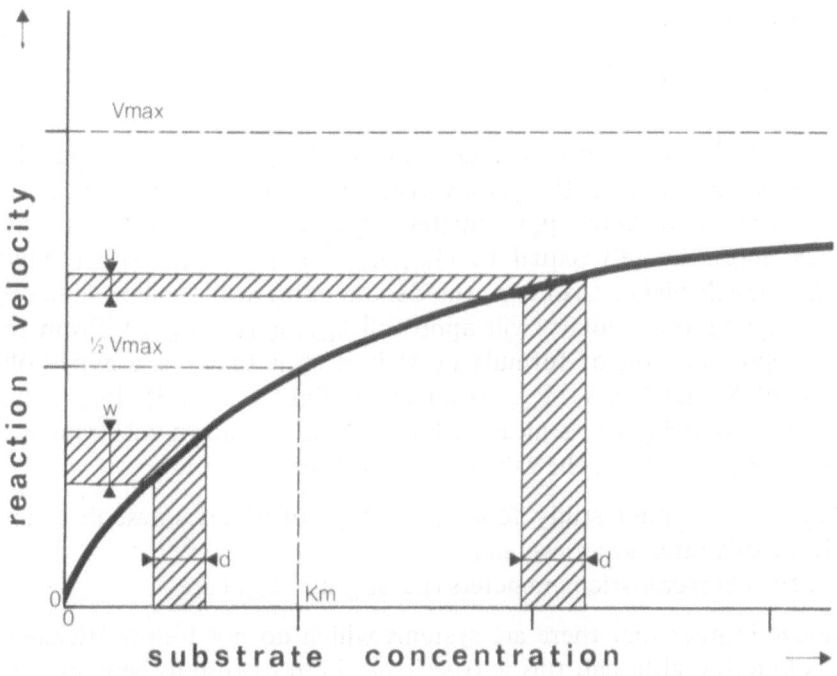

Fig. I.6. Dependence of reaction velocity on substrate consumption. A decrease in substrate concentration of *d* will cause a small decrease of reaction velocity (*u*) at high substrate concentrations but a large one (*w*) at low substrate concentrations.

of the reaction. When the amount of enzyme is to be estimated from the reaction velocity, as is usually the aim with chromogenic substrates, this decrease in substrate concentration should not bring about an appreciable decrease in reaction velocity. This can be achieved by:
1. measuring at substrate concentrations that are sufficiently high at the onset of the reaction and
2. measuring over a time lapse in which not too much of the initial substrate has been converted i.e. by measuring initial reaction rates.

This is illustrated in Fig. I.6. In order to approach this problem quantitatively, it is necessary to employ the general equation for enzymatic reaction rates known as the Michaelis-Menten formula that we will discuss presently.

I.6. The characteristic parameters of an enzymatic reaction

In practice, the relation between reaction velocity, reaction constants and enzyme and substrate concentrations is given by the so-called

Michaelis-Menten formula

$$V = \frac{k_{cat} \, E.S.}{K_m + S} \tag{1.3}$$

This formula includes both formulas previously given for low and high substrate concentrations. It is easily seen that for small values of S the denominator will become approximately equal to K_m so that the velocity becomes approximately equal to (k_{cat}/K_m). E.S. On the other hand, when S is much higher than K_m, the denominator will be approximately equal to S and the velocity will approach k_{cat}. E (i.e. V_{max}). From the graphic representation of formula (1.3) it is seen that v is a hyperbolic function of S that has a V_{max} as an upper limit (Fig. I.5). In practice the reaction velocity (v) is measured at a series of known substrate concentrations (S) and from the values obtained it can be seen

a. if the system under study follows the type of kinetics described here (Michaelis-Menten kinetics), and
b. what the characteristic parameters (i.e. K_m and k_{cat}) are.

The above implies that there are systems which do not follow Michaelis-Menten kinetics; although this is true it need not disturb us here, because most enzymatic reactions do not deviate and in the field of chromogenic substrates no exceptions to this model have been reported.

The inverse form of the Michaelis-Menten relationship is particularly useful, it leads to the following formula:

$$\frac{1}{v} = \frac{1}{k_{cat} E} + \frac{K_m}{k_{cat} E} \cdot \frac{1}{S} \tag{1.4}$$

From this it can be concluded that there is a linear relationship between $1/v$ and $1/S$ (Fig. I.7).

When in a series of measurements $1/v$ is plotted against $1/S$, a so-called Lineweaver-Burk plot is obtained. When the Michaelis-Menten formula applies, points in that plot lie on a straight line. The intercept of that line with the ordinate gives $1/V_{max}$, that with the abcissa $-1/K_m$. Usually, the experimental error leaves considerable latitude in the estimation of K_m and V_{max} in this way. As a rule of thumb, it can be said, that K_m or V_{max} have to differ by a factor two or more in order to be considered significantly different. The error in the assessment of K_m and V_{max} from experimental data can *not* be improved by making the best fit of a straight line through the experimental points with mathematical procedures for linear regression. This is because the inverse values of experimental data do not carry the same weight. The prints at the lower left hand side of the graph are determined with much more accuracy than those at the upper right hand side. Good mathematical

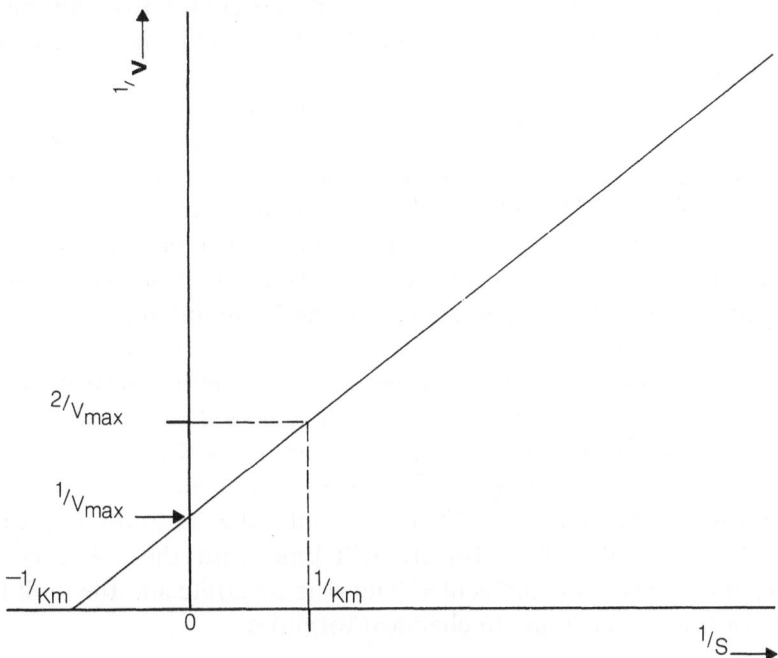

Fig. I.7. Graphic representation of the inverse of reaction velocity ($1/v$) as a function of the inverse of the substrate concentration ($1/S$): Lineweaver-Burk plot.

procedures for fitting a rectangular hyperbola should be used if such a treatment of the data is necessary (11, 17). Usually a best fit made by eye and allowing for more play of the points in the right part of the curve will be sufficient.

I.7. Enzyme inhibition

Everything that disturbs the spatial structure of a protein such as denaturing circumstances (heat, extreme pH changes, organic solvents, frothing) or extensive proteolysis will destroy its activity as well. Apart from that, specific substances may inactivate an enzyme because they react with and modify that enzyme and so prevent reaction of the enzyme with its substrate. Several types of inhibition exist. They can be divided in two groups:

a. those in which the inhibitor reacts with the active centre, and
b. those in which the inhibitor reacts with another part of the molecule but still prevents proper reaction of the active centre.

The latter type is called uncompetitive or non-competitive inhibition and will not be discussed further here. Reactions with the active centre of an enzyme are very important.

We imagine a substance (inhibitor, I) that can bind to the enzyme at the active centre like the substrate can, but that, unlike the substrate, cannot be converted into a product. Now there are two possibilities. Either the inhibitor is bound irreversibly to the active centre or it is bound reversibly. If the binding is irreversible that enzyme molecule will never again be able to catalyze a reaction. In principle as many enzyme molecules will be inactivated as there are inhibitor molecules present in the solution.

When on the other hand the binding between the inhibitor molecule and the active centre is reversible, there will exist a chemical equilibrium between the free and the inhibited form. How much there is in the free form depends on the amount of inhibitor present and the affinity of the inhibitor for the enzyme. When not only the inhibitor is present but also the substrate, the substrate will bind with the active centre of part of the free enzyme molecules. Thus the substrate and the inhibitor compete for the free enzyme. In chemical formulas

$$E + S \rightleftharpoons ES \rightarrow E + P$$
$$E + I \underset{K_i}{\rightleftharpoons} EI$$

How much enzyme is occupied in the enzyme substrate complex (ES) and hence catalytically active in producing product and how much enzyme is occupied in the enzyme inhibitor complex (EI) and hence catalytically inactive depends on the magnitude of the reaction constants and on the concentrations of each of the substances (S and I) present. At an infinite concentration of S, I will have no chance to compete and the maximal reaction velocity will result, as if no inhibitor was present. Therefore, in a case of competitive inhibition V_{max} will be always equal to V_{max} of the uninhibited reaction. K_m, however, will appear to be larger (see Fig. I.8).

I.8. Rate constants and enzymatic mechanism

The following two paragraphs are not obligatory reading for the practice of the work with chromogenic substrates. It gives part of the theoretical background of the formulas developed and can be skipped by those only interested in the practical sides of the subjects.

K_m and k_{cat} as obtained from the Lineweaver-Burk plots are the constants that quantitatively describe enzyme action when initial rates

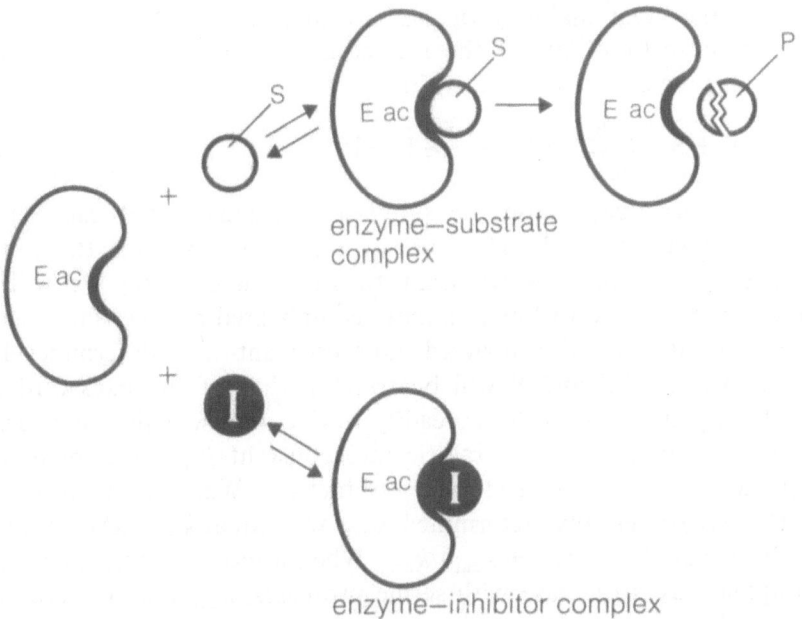

Fig. I.8. An enzymatic reaction in the presence of an inhibitor. I = inhibitor. See also Fig. I.1.

are measured under so-called steady state conditions. The reaction is said to be in a steady state when the concentration of enzyme-substrate complex(es) has built up and does no longer change with time. This means that the very first phase of the reaction during which the enzyme-substrate complex concentration rises from zero to its maximal level is neglected. This 'transient state' lasts less than one millisecond when serine proteases act on amide bonds. As the reaction is usually measured in the range of minutes, the transient state can be safely neglected and the steady state assumption can be accepted. The initial rate in fact is that rate that is obtained in the early phase of the reaction just when the enzyme-substrate complex has reached its maximal concentration. Because of the breakdown of substrate this rate is not maintained. In fact, it starts to decline as soon as it has been reached. This decline, however, is slow, and can usually be neglected during the first minutes of the reaction, at least when there is much more substrate than there is enzyme. It is therefore safe to assess the initial reaction rates on basis of the product formation in the first minutes of the reaction. It should, however, indeed be checked experimentally that the reaction rate does not decline during the measuring period (see also chapter II).

Anyhow the conditions of the 'steady state' and 'initial rate' are fulfilled in the great majority of cases. Under these conditions K_m and k_{cat} are specific functions of the rate constants that describe the mechanism of enzyme action. The most simple mechanism possible is

$$E + S \underset{k_{off}}{\overset{k_{on}}{\rightleftharpoons}} ES \xrightarrow{k_{cat}} E + P \qquad (1.5)$$

It is proper practice to use the simplest mechanism that can explain the phenomena observed. The above mechanism explains the kinetic properties of the enzymes we want to study here. Later we will see that they in fact act according to a more complicated mechanism.

The magnitude of the forward rate constant k_{on} determines how many collisions of E and S will be fruitful, that of the backward rate constant k_{off} determines how readily the complex will fall apart in enzyme and substrate. The catalytic rate constant k_{cat} determines how readily the complex will produce a product (P). When mechanism (1.5) holds the experimentally determined k_{cat} will equal k_{cat} defined above. K_m will be equal to $(k_{off} + k_{cat})/k_{on}$. When a more complicated mechanism applies, as is the case with serine proteases, k_{cat} and K_m are more complicated functions of the true rate constants.

I.9. The reaction mechanism of serine proteases

A large amount of experimental evidence obtained by other techniques than steady state kinetics made it necessary to expand our picture of the catalytic action of serine proteases considerably. A serine protease that attacks a (chromogenic) substrate first forms a complex with that substrate via noncovalent bonds. In the following a noncovalent bond will be shown by a dot ($\cdot$). The enzyme will be depicted by E$-$OH, $-$OH being the reacting group of the serine residue in the active centre. The substrate will be rendered by

$$\begin{array}{cc} O & H \\ \| & | \\ R-C-N-R' \end{array}$$

This is the vulnerable amide bond with the attached side groups. In the case of a chromogenic substrate

$$\begin{array}{c} O \\ \| \\ R-C- \end{array}$$ is the peptide part and $$\begin{array}{c} H \\ | \\ -N-R' \end{array}$$ is the paranitroanilide group.

In the first step of the reaction sequence a noncovalent enzyme-substrate complex (the Michaelis complex) is formed:

$$\text{E-OH} + \text{R-}\overset{\displaystyle O}{\overset{\|}{C}}\text{-}\overset{\displaystyle H}{\overset{|}{N}}\text{-R}' \longrightarrow \text{R-}\overset{\displaystyle O}{\overset{\|}{C}}\text{-}\overset{\displaystyle H}{\overset{|}{N}}\text{-R}'$$

$$\text{E-OH}$$

enzyme + substrate $\longrightarrow$ Michaelis complex

Internal bondshifts in the Michaelis complex cause a covalent tetrahedral complex to arise:

$$\text{R-}\overset{\displaystyle O}{\overset{\|}{C}}\text{-}\overset{\displaystyle H}{\overset{|}{N}}\text{-R}' \rightleftharpoons \text{R-}\overset{\displaystyle O^-}{\overset{|}{C}}\text{- -}\overset{\displaystyle H}{\overset{|}{N}}\text{-R}'$$

$$\text{E-OH} \qquad\qquad \text{E-O- - -H}^+$$

Michaelis complex $\rightleftharpoons$ tetrahedral complex

In the third step of the reaction, the $-C-N-$ bond is broken, giving rise to an acylenzyme intermediate and an amine product:

$$\text{R-}\overset{\displaystyle O^-}{\overset{|}{C}}\text{- - -}\overset{\displaystyle H}{\overset{|}{N}}\text{-R}' \rightleftharpoons \text{R-}\overset{\displaystyle O}{\overset{\|}{C}} \quad + \quad \overset{\displaystyle H}{\overset{|}{N}}\text{-R}'$$

$$\text{E-O- - -H}^+ \qquad\qquad \text{E-O} \qquad\qquad \text{H}$$

tetrahedral complex $\rightleftharpoons$ acylenzyme + amine (product I)

In the case of a chromogenic substrate, this amine is *p*-nitroaniline. As the third reaction is the rate determining step in the reaction sequence, the use of the coloured product *p*-nitroaniline to monitor the disappearance of the substrate is justified. In the next reactions the acylenzyme is split by a reverse of the three reactions described above. The acylenzyme reacts with a water molecule to form a tetrahedral complex.

$$\text{R-}\overset{\displaystyle O}{\overset{\|}{C}} \quad + \quad \overset{\displaystyle O\text{-H}}{} \quad\quad \text{R-}\overset{\displaystyle O^-}{\overset{|}{C}}\text{- - -O-H}$$

$$\text{E-O} \qquad\qquad \text{H} \qquad\qquad \text{E-O- - -H}^+$$

acylenzyme + water $\rightleftharpoons$ tetrahedral complex

Again internal bondshifts lead from this tetrahedral complex to a non-covalent complex:

$$
\begin{array}{ccc}
\overset{\displaystyle O^-}{\underset{\displaystyle |}{}} & & \overset{\displaystyle O}{\underset{\displaystyle \|}{}} \\
R-C\cdots O-H & \rightleftharpoons & R-C-OH \\
\vdots \quad \vdots & & \\
E-O\cdots H^+ & & E-OH
\end{array}
$$

tetrahedral complex $\rightleftharpoons$ noncovalent complex

This noncovalent complex falls apart in the free enzyme and the second product:

$$
\begin{array}{ccc}
\overset{\displaystyle O}{\underset{\displaystyle \|}{}} & & \overset{\displaystyle O}{\underset{\displaystyle \|}{}} \\
R-C-OH & \rightleftharpoons & R-C-OH \;+ E-OH \\
& & \\
E-OH & &
\end{array}
$$

noncovalent complex $\rightleftharpoons$ peptide $\quad$ + enzyme
$\qquad\qquad\qquad\qquad\quad$ (product II)

In case of a chromogenic substrate this second product is the peptide part of the substrate.

The whole process can be summarized as follows:

$$
E + S \underset{k_{-1}}{\overset{k_{+1}}{\rightleftharpoons}} ES \underset{k_{-2}}{\overset{k_{+2}}{\rightleftharpoons}} EP_2 + P_1 \underset{k_{-3}}{\overset{k_{+3}}{\rightleftharpoons}} E + P_2
$$

The relative magnitudes of the rate constants can vary appreciably between various enzyme-substrate couples. In the derivation of the steady state rate equation for serine proteases the back reactions

$(E + P_2 \overset{k_{-3}}{\to} EP_2$ and $EP_2 + P_1 \overset{k_{-2}}{\to} ES)$ can be ignored because:

a. the constants k_{-2} and k_{-3} are small, and
b. P_1 and P_2 are small in the initial phase of the reaction.

Under these conditions the reaction scheme reduces to:

$$
E + S \underset{k_{-1}}{\overset{k_{+1}}{\rightleftharpoons}} ES \overset{k_2}{\longrightarrow} EP_2 + P_1 \overset{k_3}{\longrightarrow} E + P_2
$$

Derivation of the rate expression for this simplified scheme gives:

$$
v = \frac{k_{+1} k_2 k_3 \, E.S}{k_{-1} k_3 + k_{+1} k_3 S + k_{+1} k_2 S}
$$

or written as the inverse of the velocity:

$$
\frac{1}{v} = \frac{k_2 + k_3}{k_2 k_3 \, E} + \frac{k_{-1}}{k_{+1} k_{+2} \, E.S}
$$

This expression is to be compared with the simple formula we used before:

$$\frac{1}{v} = \frac{1}{k_{cat}E} + \frac{K_m}{k_{cat}E} \cdot \frac{1}{S}$$

Comparison of both expressions for $1/v$ learns that:

$$k_{cat} = \frac{k_2 k_3}{k_2 + k_3} \quad \text{and} \quad K_m = \frac{k_{+3} k_{-1}}{k_{+1}(k_2 + k_3)}$$

With amide substrates, such as the natural protein substrates of serine proteases or chromogenic substrates, k_3 is appreciably greater than k_2. This causes that EP_2 hardly piles up and that the formation rate of P_1 pretty well reflects the formation of P_2 as well.

The situation can be easily visualized by a series of vessels through which water flows. The level of water in the vessels indicates the concentrations. The diameter of the tubes is proportional to the reaction constants and the fact that k_{-2} and k_{-3} are to be neglected is represented by the fact that no liquid from the vessels C and D can flow back to vessel B resp. C (Fig. I.9). With ester substrates like TAMe and BAMe k_3 is smaller than k_2 and an appreciable concentration of EP_2 will have to be built up before the breakdown of EP_2 will equal its formation rate. If in the model the tap k_3 is smaller than tap k_2 the level in C will rise until enough pressure is built up to ensure a steady high flux through tap k_3. The formation of P_1, being equal to the formation of EP will show an initial burst and then slow down because the amount of free enzyme (E) declines. In the ensuing steady state the level of free enzyme is replenished from the breakdown of EP in the last reaction (N.B. this situation is not adequately depicted by the hydrolic model).

When k_3 is zero all enzyme will eventually be occupied in the form of EP_2, only an initial burst of P_1 is seen. The amount of P_1 then equals the amount of enzyme initially present. The substrate then acts as an irreversible inhibitor. When P_1 can be conveniently measured such a substrate can be used as an active site titrant (see paragraph I.12 for a further treatment).

Natural polypeptide inhibitors like soybean trypsin inhibitor (SBTI) act by a slightly different mechanism. There P_2 remains attached to E so that no free enzyme is restored. Kinetically this situation is equivalent to EP_2 being stable.

All these relations are of interest to the enzymologist only; in practice k_{cat} and K_m can be used as they come and provide sufficient information for dealing with the situations encountered. In general k_{cat} will be smaller than any of the forward rate constants after formation of the enzyme-substrate complex and mechanistically it can best be envisaged as the

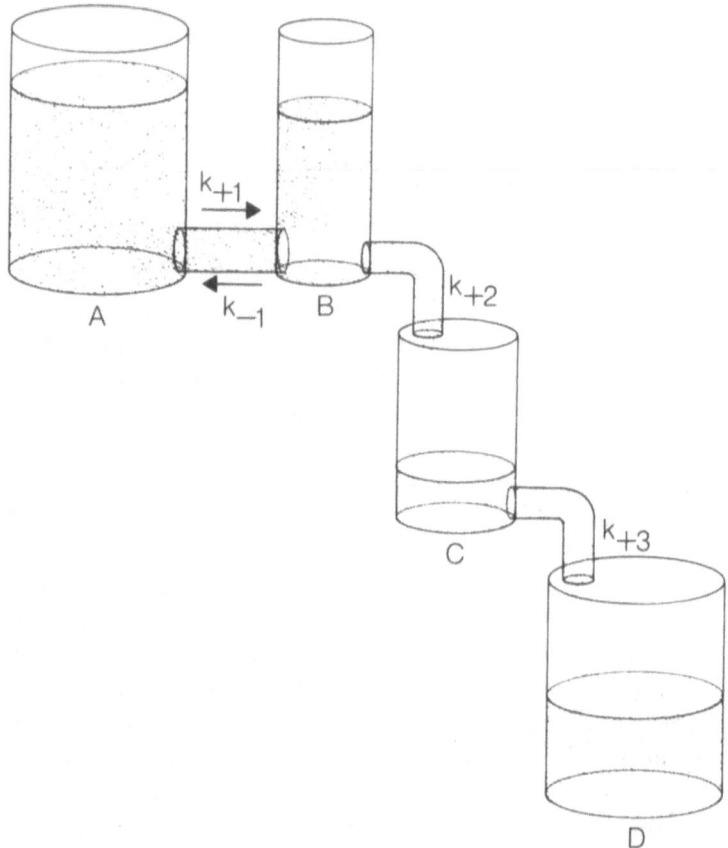

Fig. I.9.   A hydraulic model of the breakdown of an amide substrate by a serine protease.

turnover number, the number of substrate molecules converted per molecule of enzyme per second. K_m is simply the substrate concentration at which half of the enzyme occurs in its bound form. A high K_m therefore will occur with an enzyme and a substrate that will not readily combine, whereas a low K_m means that enzyme and substrate combine eagerly.

As already indicated above, k_{cat}/K_m is a measure of the efficiency of the enzyme. In practice, it represents the rate constant of the combination of substrate with free enzyme and is a useful parameter when analysing situations where competing enzymes and substrates occur.

I.10. Transient state kinetics

Transient state kinetics are not of great importance for the situations where chromogenic substrates are usually employed. They will therefore be mentioned only briefly. During a short period after mixing of enzyme and substrate, the enzyme-substrate complex will be formed faster than it is broken down. This lasts until its concentration is so high that its breakdown, the velocity of which is proportional to the concentration, equals its formation rate. With serine proteases and amide substrates, it takes less than 1 millisecond to approach the steady state.

This lapse of time is called presteady state or transient state. By special techniques the reaction rates in such short time spans can be measured. It is then seen that the steady state velocity is reached as an exponential function. From the parameters of this function some of the individual true rate constants like k_{+1} can be assessed. The interested reader is further referred to texts on general enzymology and the specialized literature (see refs. 1–10).

I.11. Data from a reaction going to completion

Theoretically the splitting of a chromogenic substrate by a serine protease will not go to completion, because the enzyme can also catalyse the back reaction, i.e., the synthesis of the chromogenic substrate from the tri-peptide and p-nitroaniline. Preliminary results from our laboratory indicate that, if not all, at least 99% of the substrate is split under standard conditions at pH values around 8 (see chapter III). For all practical purposes the reaction can be considered to go to completion. When a reaction is allowed to go to completion all substrate will be used. As the reaction velocity is a function of substrate concentration, it will decrease during the reaction. At any moment, the reaction velocity v_t will be equal to the velocity that can be calculated to belong to the then prevailing substrate concentration S_t

$$v_t = \frac{V_{max} S_t}{K_m + S_t} \tag{1.6}$$

By integration of this formula the product concentration as a function of time can be found. The ensuing formula is

$$V_{max} \cdot t = P_t + K_m \ln \frac{S_0}{S_0 - P_t} \tag{1.7}$$

where t = time (in seconds) since the beginning of the reaction

S_0 = substrate concentration at the onset

P_t = product concentration at time t.

This is a relatively awkward formula that can be transformed into a handy form.

Therefore, we first introduce two new variables x and y so that

$$x = \left(\ln \frac{S_0}{S_0 - P_t} \right) \Big/ t \qquad (1.8)$$

and

$$y = P_t / t$$

then

$$y = V_{max} - K_m \cdot x \qquad (1.9)$$

and a plot of y against x will be a straight line that has $- K_m$ as a slope and V_{max} as an intercept with the ordinate.

The evident advantage is that the kinetic parameters K_m and V_{max} are obtained from one experiment only. There are, however, several drawbacks. For small P_t's x will be near zero and y will hardly vary. For high P_t's $(Pt \rightarrow S_0)$ the experimental error in x will be large. A computer program has been prepared that carries out the calculations shown and that also gives an estimate of the error in the constants obtained (12).

I.12. Active site titration

A. Principles

The following describes in some detail active site titration, a technique that hardly will become common practice in the coagulation laboratory. It is an important technique to characterise pure enzymes and obtain valid kinetic constants. It can not be carried out in patient samples because it needs high amounts of pure material. Because of its importance in defining the system we are working with and because of the insight it gives in the essentials of working with enzymes we will discuss it here.

Subtile changes in primary or tertiary structure, often not detectable by the usual physical and chemical criteria of homogeneity can cause profound changes in the activity of an enzyme molecule. A serine protease sample that has been purified so as to meet the criteria of homogeneity will usually not consist entirely of molecules that have identical catalytic activity. It is possible that a fraction of the molecules is inactive. When e.g. bovine factor VII is purified in the presence of proteolytic inhibitors (e.g. DFP) in order to prevent its breakdown, part of the factor VII molecules will react with the inhibitor and a 'dead' molecule that by all practical physico-chemical means will be indistinguishable from the intact ones, will be present in the preparation. It will not count in an active site titration, however. The same effect can be – and in practice often is – caused by partial denaturation.

Active site titration is a kinetic means to assess the amount of active enzyme molecules in a mixed population of otherwise indistinguishable material. This is done by substances called active site titrants. In principle, these are substrates that are handled by the enzyme according to the general formula:

$$E + S \underset{k_{-1}}{\overset{k_{+1}}{\rightleftharpoons}} ES \overset{k_2}{\longrightarrow} EP_2 + P_1 \overset{k_3}{\longrightarrow} E + P_2 \qquad (1.10)$$

Only with these substrates k_3 is much smaller than k_2 or even zero. When k_3 is zero, and P_1 is a product that can be measured e.g. spectrophotometrically or fluorimetrically, for each molecule of active enzyme one molecule of P_1 will be formed and the amount of coloured molecules that develops is equal to the amount of active enzyme (Fig. I.10a). Usually k_3 will not be zero so that after an initial burst of colour there will be a continuous steady colour production (Fig. I.10b). In that case analysis of the curve obtained can still give the amount of active sites. We will now first give the theory of active site titration and then a practical example. (For further information see refs. 25–30.)

B. Theory

As shown by Bender et al. (13) the rate of P_1 production is given by the following formula:

$$P_1 = At + \pi (1 - e^{-bt}) \qquad (1.11)$$

where

$$A = \frac{k_{cat} E_0 S_0}{K_m + S_0} \qquad k_{cat} = \frac{k_2 \cdot k_3}{k_2 + k_3} \qquad (1.12)$$

$$\pi = E_0 \left[\frac{k_2/(k_2 + k_3)}{1 + K_m/S_0} \right]^2 \qquad (1.13)$$

When the transient phase is over, e^{-bt} approaches zero so that in the steady state the product formation is given by

$$P_1 = At + \pi \qquad (1.14)$$

When $k_2 \gg k_3$, the squared term in formula (1.12) will approach unity and hence π will approach E_0. If this is not the case, π has to be determined at several substrate concentrations. Then a plot of $1/\sqrt{\pi}$ versus

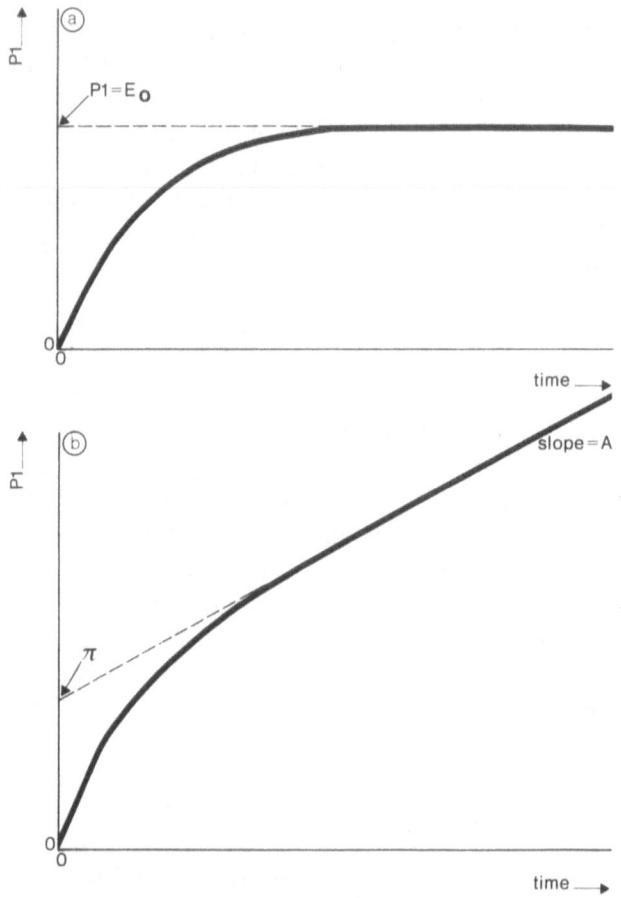

Fig. I.10. Active site titration. a) above: when the acyl enzyme is not broken down ($k_3 = 0$); b) below: when the acyl enzyme is broken down slowly ($k_3 \neq 0; k_3 < k_2$).

$1/S_0$ will intercept the ordinate at $1/\sqrt{E_0}$. This follows from a rearrangement of formula (1.13):

$$\frac{1}{\sqrt{\pi}} = \frac{k_2 + k_3}{k_2} \cdot \frac{1}{\sqrt{E_0}} + \frac{(k_2 + k_3) \cdot k_m}{k_2 \cdot \sqrt{E_0}} \cdot \frac{1}{S_0} \tag{1.15}$$

C. Practice

A practical example will be taken from Lindhout *et al.* (1978). The titration of activated factor X was performed according to Smith (1973). Microcuvettes in which $300\,\mu l$ of solution could be measured at 1 cm wavelength were used. In a typical experiment $150\,\mu g$ factor X_a in $300\,\mu l$ 0.1 M sodium barbital buffer pH 8.3 was added in the sample cuvette. The reference cuvette contained the same volume of buffer solution alone. To both cuvettes $3\,\mu l$ of a 0.01 M solution of p-Nitro-phenyl-p'-guanidinobenzoate hydrochloride (NPGB) was added simultaneously. The reaction was followed at 410 nm in an Aminco DW-2 spectrophotometer at 25°C. E_{410} for p-nitrophenol, the product of splitting of NPGB, was calculated to be 17 500 under these conditions. In this way a trace like in Fig. I.10b was obtained.

A list of active site titrants, that have been used for various serine proteases, is found in Table I.1. Attention should be paid to the fact that k_{+2} and k_{+3} are dependent upon pH; k_{+3} that may be conveniently small at one pH and may be high at another, in this way making active site titration impracticable.

We dwell relatively long upon this subject, because exact knowledge of the amount of active sites is of prime importance for the determination of k_{cat}. From Lineweaver-Burk plots $V_{max} = k_{cat} \cdot E$ is obtained, so E has to be known in order to know k_{cat}. In enzyme preparations that are homogeneous by all usual criteria, up to 50% of the molecules can be in an inactive form. Substituting the amount of enzyme added for the amount of active enzyme can therefore lead to important errors.

I.13. Simultaneous reactions in complicated reaction mixtures

Chromogenic substrates are usually not so specific that they can be split by only one enzyme. Determinations of coagulation factors etc. often are carried out in complex mixtures in which more than one active enzyme can be present. Also the natural substrates of these enzymes usually will be present in the reaction mixture. It is therefore of practical importance to investigate the kinetic consequences of the simultaneous presence of two enzymes and/or two substrates.

A. Two substrates and one enzyme

We remember that the reaction velocity of an enzymatic reaction is a simple function of the amount of free enzyme present (i.e. not counting those molecules occupied in an enzyme-substrate complex).

$$v = k_{cat}/K_m \, E_{free} \cdot S \qquad (1.16)$$

This formula will hold irrespective of the enzyme in its bound form being bound to one or two substrates. When two substrates are present, the ratio of the velocities of the breakdown of each substrate is easily calculated to be

$$R = v/v^* = ((k_{cat}/K_m)S_1)/((k_{cat}^*/K_m^*)S_2) \qquad (1.17)$$

Table I.1.   List of active site titrants for several serine proteases (refs. 21–26).

Enzyme(s)	Active site titrant
α-chymotrypsin	2-hydroxy-*p*-nitro-α-toluenesulfonic acid sulfone (spectrophotometric determination)
α-chymotrypsin	trans-cinnamoyl imidazole (spectrophotometric determination)
α-chymotrypsin	*p*-nitrophenyl acetate (spectrophotometric determination)
α-chymotrypsin	*p*-nitrophenyl trimethylacetate (spectrophotometric determination)
α-chymotrypsin	*p*-nitrophenyl N-benzyloxycarbonyl-L-tyrosinate (spectrophotometric determination)
α-chymotrypsin	*p*-nitrophenyl N-acetyl-DL-tryptophanate (spectrophotometric determination)
α-chymotrypsin	4-methylumbelliferyl-(N,N,N-triethylammonium) cinnamate (fluormetric determination)
α-chymotrypsin	4-methylumbelliferyl *p*- ω-dimethylsulfonioaceta-midobenzoate (fluorimetric determination)
trypsin	*p*-nitrophenyl-N^2-acetyl-N^1-benzylcarbazate (spectrophotometric determination)
trypsin	*p*-nitrophenyl-*p*′-amidinobenzoate HCl (spectrophotometric determination)
trypsin	N^α-methyl-N^α-toluenesulfonyl-L-lysine β-naphtyl-ester (originally reported as spectrophotometric determination, easily adapted for fluorometric determination)
trypsin	diisopropylphosphofluoridate (DFP) (radiometric determination)
trypsin	1-chloro-3-tosylamido-7-aminoheptane (TLCK) (spectrophotometric determination)
trypsin	ethyl-*p*-guanidinobenzoate (spectrophotometric determination)
trypsin	*p*-nitrophenyl ethyl diazomalonate (spectrophotometric determination)
trypsin, thrombin	*p*-nitrophenyl N^α-benzyloxycarbonyl-L-lysinate HCl (spectrophotometric determination)
trypsin, plasma kallikrein, plasmin (good), thrombin, factor X_a (less satisfactory)	*p*-nitrophenyl-*p*′-guanidinobenzoate HCl (*p*-NPGB) (spectrophotometric determination)
α- and β-trypsin, thrombin, factor X_a, human plasmin, human plasma kallikrein, boar acrosin	methylumbelliferyl *p*-guanidinobenzoate (fluorimetric determination
thrombin	N-benzyloxycarbonyl-L-tyrosine *p*-nitrophenylester (spectrophotometric determination)
thrombin	N-benzyloxycarbonly-L-lysine-*p*-nitrophenylester (spectrophotometric determination)

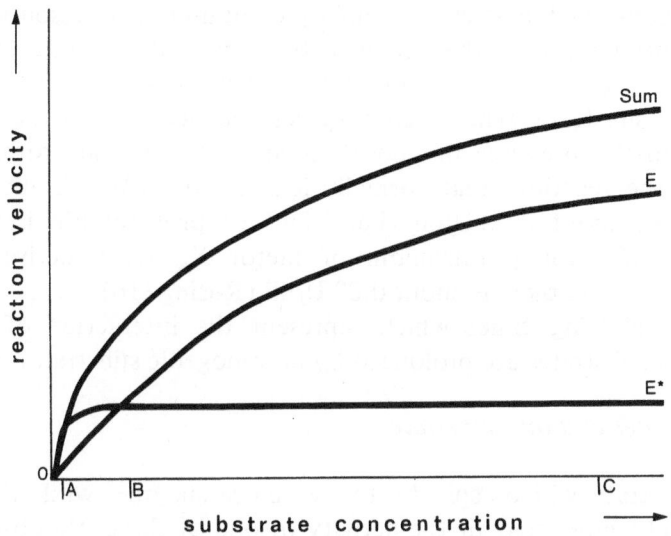

Fig. I.11. Two enzymes acting on one substrate (see text).

(the asterisks denote the symbols pertaining to the second substrate). The ratio is independent of the amount of enzyme but dependent upon the concentration of the substrates present and their efficiency constants. When a chromogenic substrate and a natural substrate are present simultaneously, the generation of one product is measured and the other substrate will act as a competitive inhibitor of that generation. The velocity observed is then:

$$v = \frac{k_{cat} E.S_1}{S_1 + K_m (1 + S_2/K_m^*)} \quad \text{for the chromogenic substrate.}$$

When, as in the case illustrated in Fig. I.11, the second substrate is also a chromogenic substrate, its splitting will add to the general colour production. The velocity of the splitting of the second substrate is simply given by the formula analogous to the one above:

$$v^* = \frac{k_{cat}^* E.S_2}{S_2 + K_m^* (1 + S_1/K_m)}$$

The decrease of the velocity of the splitting of the first substrate brought about by the competition of the second can be substantially larger than the increase in the overall velocity by the splitting of the second substrate.

From the fact that the observed velocity equals the sum of the individual rates ($v_{obs} = v + v^*$) and the fact that the formulas for v and v^* are known, S_1 can be calculated in such cases when all reaction constants and S_2 are known (and vice versa). The necessary arithmetic is simple but cumbersome and best carried out by computer. The lesson we learn in the meantime is that the presence of a natural substrate (say pro-thrombin for factor X_a) may inhibit the reaction of an enzyme with a chromogenic substrate. When factor X_a is to be measured by the splitting of S 2222 in the presence of phospholipid, factor V and prothrombin, the K_m of the reaction, that normally is about 0.3 mM, will increase to 1.0 mM when about 0.08 U/ml (i.e. 1.8%) of prothrombin is present, because the K_m for prothrombin of factor X_a when active in the prothrombinase complex, is about 0.03 U/ml (Rosing (16)).

Inversely, clotting times which represent the interaction of natural enzymes and substrates are prolonged by chromogenic substrates.

B. Two enzymes and one substrate

Often a substrate will be split by two or more enzymes while the inves-tigator is only interested in the activity of one of these. He observes an overall reaction velocity (v_{total}), but wants to know only that velocity that is of interest to him. It therefore is useful to be able to calculate the quotient $v_{interest}/v_{total}$.

When two enzymes compete for one substrate and yield the same product, it can be easily calculated that for each of the enzymes holds

$$v = \frac{k_{cat}.E.S}{K_m + S} \tag{1.18}$$

When the symbols v, k_{cat}, K_m, and E are defined to belong to the one enzyme and v^*, k_{cat}^*, K_m^* and E^* to the other, the ratio of the velocities is found to be:

$$v/v^* = E/E^* \cdot \frac{k_{cat}(K_m^* + S)}{k_{cat}^*(K_m + S)} \tag{1.19}$$

This is a relatively awkward formula that does not allow immediate insight in the situation but that can be used to calculate whether a con-taminating enzyme will be disturbing or not when the kinetic constants and the substrate concentrations are known. When it appears that an enzyme will be disturbing still it is possible to calculate the contribution of one enzyme to the overall observed rate. Again cumbersome calcu-lations are necessary that are best left to a computer.

Anyhow, to estimate the relative contribution of different enzymes to substrate breakdown, it is absolutely necessary to have a good estimate of the kinetic constants involved. It is not sufficient to know the relative rates at one fixed substrate concentration only. Unfortunately this type of information is often the only one available in the literature.

We can also approach this problem in a more intuitive way. Fig. 1.11

shows the substrate dependence of reaction velocity for two different enzymes. The one (E) with a high maximal velocity $(V_{\text{max}} = k_{\text{cat}}. E)$, the other (E^*) with a low V_{max} $(V^*_{\text{max}} = k^*_{\text{cat}}. E^*)$. The one with the high V_{max} is assumed to have a high K_m as well. It is easily seen that at substrate concentration A, predominantly enzyme E^* is measured, at concentration B, both enzymes contribute equally and at concentration C, enzyme E plays the main role. The sum of the velocities will not be a simple hyperbola. This also indicates the way to diagnose whether in practice two enzymes are acting or one. With two enzymes, the Lineweaver-Burk plot will not be straight precisely because the S-v plot is not a hyperbola. It should be stressed that there are many other reasons for Lineweaver-Burk plots not to be straight.

References

A. General texts on enzymes and enzyme kinetics. This selection is arbitrary, based on the author's experience. Many more useful texts may exist.

1. Biophysical Chemistry. Bloomfield VA, Harrington RE (eds.). Freeman and Co., San Francisco (Readings from Scientific American), 1975, pp. 118–154
2. The Enzymes, Vol. 1 and 2. Boyer PD (ed.). Academic Press, New York, 1970. Very extensive advanced text
3. Organic Chemistry of Life, Calvin M, Prior WA (eds.). Freeman and Co., San Francisco (Readings from Scientific American), 1973, Chapter 35. Neurath H: Protein digesting enzymes
4. Enzymes. Dixon M, Webb EC, Longman, London, 1971 Chapters 4, 8, 10 Classical advanced text
5. Enzyme Structure and Mechanism. Fersht A. WH Freeman and Co., San Francisco, 1977. Extremely useful text
6. Kurzes Lehrbuch der Biochemie. Karlsson P. G. Thieme Verlag, Stuttgart, 1980. Chapter 5. Students text
7. Biochemistry. Lehninger AL. Worth Publ. Inc., New York, 1975. Chapters 6, 8 and 9. Student text
8. Kinetics of Chemical and Enzyme-Catalyzed Reactions. Piszxiewicz D. Oxford University Press, New York, 1977. Short advanced text
9. Enzyme Kinetics. Segel IH. Wiley Intersci., New York, 1975. Extensive advanced text
10. Kinetics of Enzyme Mechanisms. Tze-Fei Wong J. Academic Press, London, 1975. Short advanced text

B. Further references

11. Wilkinson GN: Biochem J 80:324–332 (1961)
12. Willems GM, Hemker HC: FEBS Letters 24:293–296 (1972)
13. Bender ML, Begué-Canton ML, Blakely RL, Brubacher LJ, Feder J, Gunter CR, Kezdy FJ, Killheffer JV, Marchall TH, Miller CG, Roeske RW, Stoops JK: J Am Chem Soc 88:5890–5896 (1966)
14. Lindhout MJ, Kop-Klaassen BHM, Hemker HC: Biochim Biophys Acta 533: 342–354 (1978)

15. Smith RL: J Biol Chem 248:2418−2423 (1973)
16. Rosing J, Tans G, Govers-Riemslag JWP, Zwaal RFA, Hemker HC: J Biol Chem 255:274−283 (1980)
17. Cornish-Bowden A, Eisenthal R: Biochem J 139:721−730 (1974)
18. Bajusz S, Barabas E, Toinsy P, Szell E, Rady D: Int J Peptide Protein Res 12: 217−221 (1978)
19. Geratz JD: Thrombosis et Diathesis Haemorrh 23:486−499 (1970)
20. Haustmann J, Markwardt E, Walsmann P: Thromb Res 12:735−744 (1978)
21. Kerdy FJ, Kaiser ET: In Methods in Enzymology. Vol. XIX. Perlmann GE, Lorand L (eds.). Academic Press, New York, 1970, pp 3−20
22. Chase Jr. T, Shaw E: In Methods in Enzymology. Vol. XIX. Perlmann GE, Lorand L (eds). Academic Press, New York, 1970, pp 20−27
23. Lundblad RL, Kingdon HS, Mann KG: In Methods in Enzymology. Vol XLV. Lorand L (ed). Academic Press, New York, 1976, pp 156−176
24. Coleman PL, Latham Jr. HG, Shaw EN: In Methods in Enzymology. Vol. XLV. Lorand L (ed). Academic Press, New York, 1976, pp 12−26
25. Walsh KA: In Methods in Enzymology. Vol. XIX. Perlmann GE, Lorand L (eds). Academic Press, New York, 1970, pp 41−63
26. Wong SC, Shaw E: Arch Biochem Biophys 161:536−543 (1974)

II. Measuring the conversion of a chromogenic substrate

Summary

In this chapter the theoretical background of and practical considerations on the measuring of reactions with chromogenic substrates are given. Paragraphs 1, 2 and 3 discuss theory and practise of spectrophotometric assay methods. The influence of temperature is considered in paragraph 4. Paragraphs 5 and 6 give general observations on the features of the reaction medium that determine the reaction velocity measured. Paragraphs 7 and 8 discuss how the experiments are best carried out in practise.

II.1. Photometric assays

Fig. II.1 shows the absorption spectrum of chromozym TH as well as that of the products obtained by thrombin catalyzed cleavage of the Arg-pNA bond to separate the peptide part from the *p*-nitroaniline. Such spectra are caused by the fact that certain chemical structures preferentially absorb light of a specific wavelength and therefore display an absorption maximum at that wavelength. A change in chemical structure brings about a change of the absorption maximum. *P*-nitroaniline has an absorption maximum at 380 nm whereas the *p*-nitroanilide group when bound to a peptide as e.g. in Chromozym TH absorbs at 323 nm (Fig. II.1). Because the absorption is a property of the molecule, its extent is proportional to the number of molecules. This property is used in the spectrophotometric measurement of concentrations. In mixtures of split and unsplit Chromozym TH the spectrum is the sum of the spectra of the two components which is seen as the gradual decrease of absorption at the 323 nm maximum and increase of absorption at the 380 nm maximum. This is illustrated in Fig. II.2. This phenomenon can be used to follow the reaction of substrate breakdown quantitatively by means of a spectrophotometer. This can be done in several ways that will be treated after the general principles of photometric assays have been discussed.

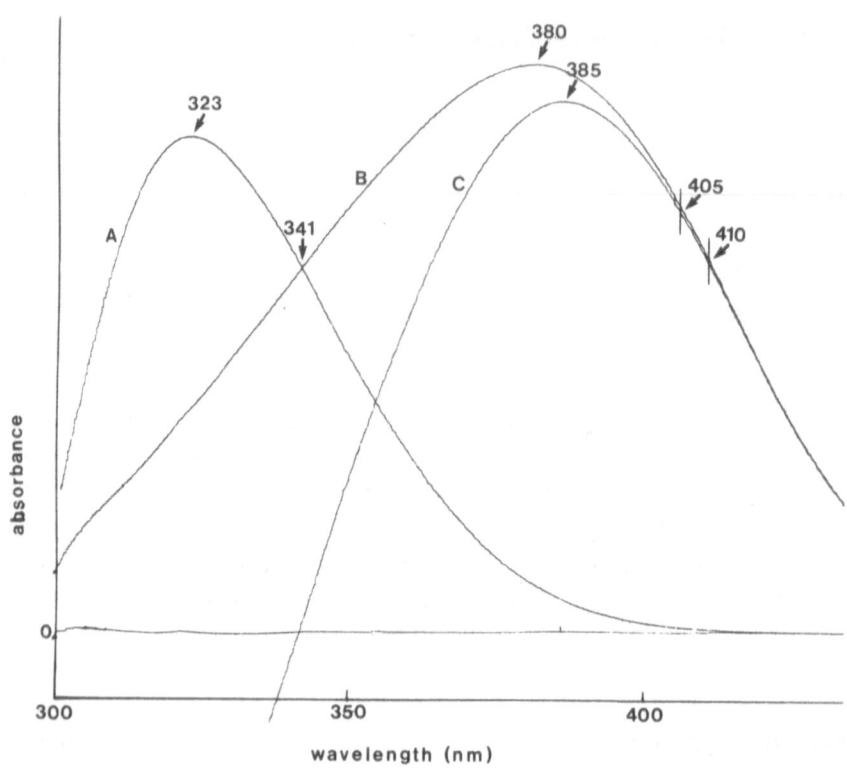

Fig. II.1. Spectra of Chromozym TH and its split products. A. Absorption spectrum of chromozym TH. N.B. the position of the peak may differ slightly in different substrates. B. Absorption spectrum of the split products of chromozym TH which is mainly due to *p*-nitroaniline. C. The difference spectrum of *A* and *B*. The figures indicate the wavelengths.

II.2. Absorption spectrophotometry

Absorption spectrophotometry is governed by Lambert-Beer's law, which relates the attenuation of light by absorbing solutions to the thickness of the layer and the concentration of the absorbing substance. For the symbols used see Table II.1. The law first defines absorbance (A) as the logarithm of the ratio of the power (intensity) of a light beam before (P_0) and after (P) passing through a solution: $A = \log(P_0/P)$. It then states that absorbance at a specific wavelength (λ) in a solution that contains a substance absorbing light of that wavelength, is proportional to the thickness of the layer through which the light passes (b) and the concentration (c) of the substance in solution, i.e. the number of molecules the light meets when passing through the solution.

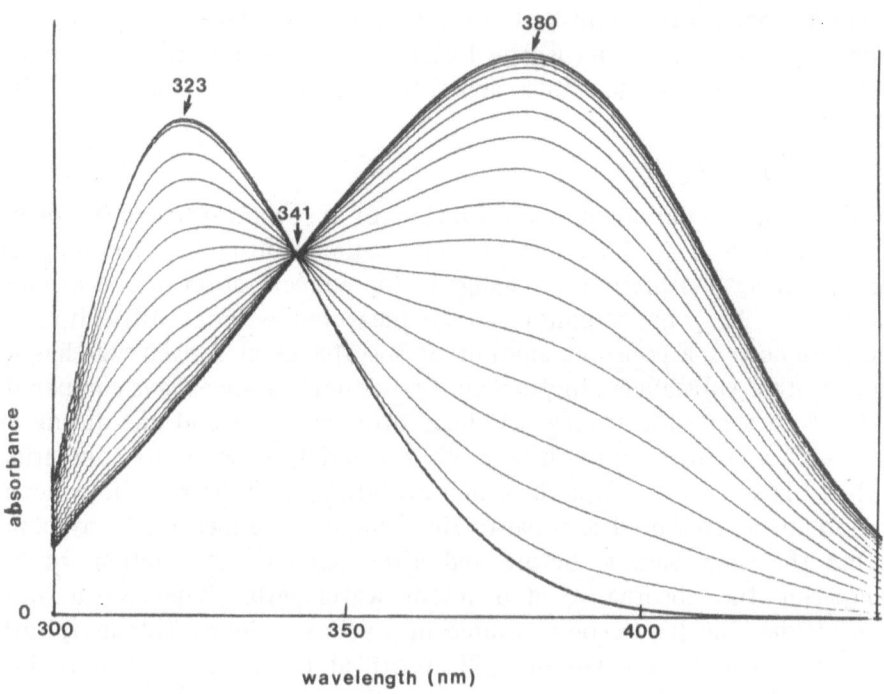

Fig. II.2. Spectra during the conversion of Chromozym TH. To 0.05 M of chromozym TH a small amount of thrombin was added and every two minutes a spectrum was recorded.

Table II.1. Units and symbols in spectrophotometry.

Accepted symbol	Definition	Accepted name	Alternatives
P	—	Power (of radiation)	I, Intensity
P_0	—	Power (or unabsorbed radiation)	I_0, Intensity
T	P/P_0	Transmittance	Transmission
A	$\log_{10} P_0/P$	Absorbance	D, Optical density E, extinction
a	$A/b \cdot c$	Absorbtivity	k, extinction coefficient, absorbancy index
b	—	Length of path	l, d
C	M/l	Molar concentration	c', % (w/v)
ϵ	A/bM	Molar absorbtivity	a_M, molecular extinction coefficient, molar absorbancy index

The proportionality constant is the absorbance obtained at the specific wavelength at unit length (usually 1 cm) and a concentration of one molar (1 M). This is called the molar absorbtivity at the wavelength ϵ_λ^{1cm}. In formula:

$$A = \epsilon_\lambda \cdot b \cdot c \tag{2.1}$$

In solution, an unknown concentration of a specific substance can be measured $(c = A/\epsilon_\lambda \cdot 1/b)$ provided no other substance absorbing at that wavelength is present. A change in the concentration of one specific substance (like p-nitroaniline) can be measured without difficulties in the presence of a constant amount of absorbance at a given wavelength due to other substances. In practice, two situations are always compared, one before a specific change has been brought about and one during or after such a change. This can be done in a variety of ways: by comparing with a blank (i.e. a sample in which everything but the specific concentration to be measured is equal to the sample to be measured); by comparing the same sample before and after starting the reaction; or by comparing the absorbance at different wavelengths. When an amount of p-nitroaniline has to be measured in a yellow solution (plasma), both the solution and p-nitroaniline will absorb at the same wavelength. The yellow colour of the plasma will hopefully remain constant during the reaction:

$$A_{total} = A_{plasma} + A_a \qquad \Delta A = \epsilon_{\lambda a} \cdot \Delta c_a \tag{2.2a}$$

$$A_{total} = \epsilon_{\lambda pl} c_{pl} + \epsilon_{\lambda a} \cdot c_a \qquad (b = 1) \tag{2.2b}$$

(subscript pl: plasma; a: addition).

In the instrument $A = \epsilon_{\lambda pl} c_{pl}$ can be set to zero. Consequently only $\Delta A = \epsilon_{\lambda a} \cdot \Delta c_a$ is measured either by setting to zero the sample at $t = 0$ or by taking as a blank a reference cuvette without substrate.

When a reaction substrate $(s) \rightarrow$ product (p) is to be measured at a wavelength where both substrate and product absorb, both contribute to the extinction.

$$A_{total} = A_{substr.} + A_{product} \tag{2.3a}$$

$$A_{total} = \epsilon_{\lambda s} \cdot c_s + \epsilon_{\lambda p} \cdot c_p \tag{2.3b}$$

The change in extinction (ΔA) with a given change in concentrations (Δc) by conversion of s into p then will be

$$\Delta A = (\epsilon_{\lambda p} - \epsilon_{\lambda s}) \Delta c \tag{2.4}$$

There will be a maximal change of extinction at that wavelength where $|\epsilon_{\lambda p} - \epsilon_{\lambda s}|$ is maximal. There will be no change where $\epsilon_{\lambda p} = \epsilon_{\lambda s}$, i.e. at the so-called 'isosbestic point' (Fig. II.2).

Table II.2.   Ratio of molar absorbtivities at different wavelength.

λ(mM)	380 a	380 Δ	385 Δ	405 Δ	410 Δ
380 a*	1.00	1.088	1.07	1.33	1.52
380 Δ	0.919	1.00	0.985	1.22	1.40
385 Δ	0.934	1.015	1.00	1.24	1.42
405 Δ	0.751	0.817	0.805	1.00	1.14
410 Δ	0.665	0.717	0.706	0.877	1.00

*This table gives the molar absorbtivities (ϵ) of p-nitroaniline at different wavelengths relative to the ϵ at another wavelength. a indicates that p-nitroaniline is measured against water. $\epsilon \approx 1.30 \times 10^4$ ($b = 1$ cm) in that case. Δ indicates that pNA is measured against a substrate solution of the same concentration, which also is the case in practice. It is seen that measuring at 385 nm increases the signal by more than 40% compared to measurement at 410 nm. At the often used wavelength of 405 nm $\epsilon = 9.92 \times 10^3$. At the isosbestic point $\epsilon = 8.27 \times 10^3$.

It is important to obtain a maximal signal from a given concentration change. This will cause a maximal sensitivity and also the signal to noise ratio will be maximal. Therefore, a spectrophotometric measurement is best carried out at a peak in the product-substrate difference spectrum. This has the additional advantage that small involuntary changes in the wavelength chosen will not lead to large changes in molar absorbtivity

$$\left(\frac{d\epsilon}{d\lambda} \approx 0 \quad \text{near the top} \right).$$

This is particularly important with grating or prism monochromators because these instruments allow a selection from a continuous spectrum and thereby introduce some latitude in determination of the wavelength at which the measurement is carried out. With filter monochromators, that usually select a line from a Hg spectrum, the wavelength may be chosen besides the peak because it lies at a fixed point not dependent upon the instrument setting.

The molar absorbtivity varies with the wavelength and at each wavelength the proper molar extinction should be used (Table II.2). When the nonspecific absorption or the scattering in the sample do vary during the experiment, as e.g. is the case in clotting plasma, it can be accounted for if this change occurs in the blank to a comparable extent. When this is not the case, one has to resort to dual wavelength techniques. The dual wavelength technique is particularly useful when measuring in turbid media and especially in media where the turbidity changes during the experiment. The principle is that one compares the change in absorbance at the isosbestic point ($\epsilon_{\lambda p} - \epsilon_{\lambda s} = 0$) and at a nearby peak in the difference spectrum of product and substrate ($|\epsilon_{\lambda p} - \epsilon_{\lambda s}|$ is maximal).

Fluctuations in light intensity, turbidity changes and some types of non-specific absorbance changes (dilution) will be equal or almost equal for both wavelengths and will therefore not be recorded by the instrument provided that indeed the two wavelengths are not far apart. If there are differences in absorbance between two wavelengths, these may still be due to non-specific effects. Turbidity e.g. will cause more scattering at shorter wavelengths than at longer ones etc. but as a rule in dual wavelength measurement these effects are negligible.

With all spectrophotometric experiments a possible source of error lies in the fact that Lambert-Beer's law holds for monochromatic light only whereas a prism- or grating monochromator does not produce ideal monochromatic light. As long as the bandwidth is small compared to the peak in the difference spectrum this will not play an important role, however. Anyhow, the bandwidth has to be specified when accurate measurements are required.

In modern instruments, 3 nm is a reasonable bandwidth. This indeed is small compared to the absorption peak of p-nitroaniline, the width of which at half maximal intensity is 84 nm.

II.3. Choice of wavelength and absorbancy range

Fig. II.1 shows the spectrum of a chromogenic substrate before (A) and after (B) splitting as well as the difference spectrum between the two (C). It is seen that 385 nm is the top of the difference spectrum and therefore is the best wavelength at which to measure concentration changes. The isosbestic point is at 341 nm so for dual wavelength measurements this is the reference wavelength of choice.

Table II.2 gives a list of wavelengths with their molar absorption coefficients for p-nitroaniline.

As to the choice of absorbance range, one is usually not free, but restricted by the chemical system under study. It can be shown from theory that spectrophotometric determinations are most accurate in the range between $A = 0.080$ and $A = 0.800$. When the chemical system allows, it is best to adapt it so that this range is covered in the experiment (see ref. 4). Because of optical limitations some spectrophotometers may give nonlinear responses at $A > 1.0$. The absorbance of p-nitroaniline is linear with the concentration from about $1-200\,\mu$mol/l (roughly $0.010-2.0$ A) in water and in 0.05 ml/l Tris buffer pH 8.0 I 0.15.

Plasma (10% v/v) in a pNA solution will decrease the absorbance by about 2%, serum (10% v/v) by less than 1% and albumin (1% w/v) urine (50% v/v) by less than 0.5%. No shifts in the location of absorbance peaks were recorded under these conditions (P. Friberger, personal communication).

The three most popular wavelengths used for the measurement of

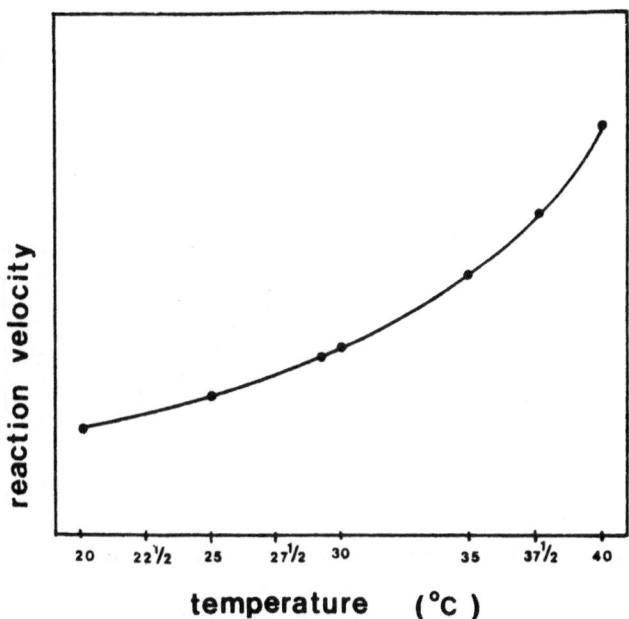

Fig. II.3. Schematic representation of the temperature dependence of the splitting of a chromogenic substrate.

p-nitroaniline are 380, 405 and 410 nm; 380 nm is the absorbancy maximum of the product, 405 and 410 nm are two wavelengths for which commercial filters are available and where the substrate does not absorb for more than 1%. The ideal wavelength, however, would be 385 nm, since the signal there is 1.42 × that at 405 nm and hence the signal to noise ratio will be better there. Lower concentration changes can thus be measured. The fact that the substrate does absorb to some extent at this wavelength in this respect is of no importance, as can be readily understood from the theory given in paragraph 2 of this chapter.

II.4. Temperature

Like all chemical reactions the velocity of the splitting of chromogenic substrates is temperature-dependent (see ref. 5). Fig. II.3 shows an example of this temperature dependance. On the basis of theoretical considerations as can be found in the general references, it can be demonstrated that each of the kinetic constants (k) of a reaction will depend upon the temperature according to the following formula:

$$\log k = -a1/T + b \qquad (2.5)$$

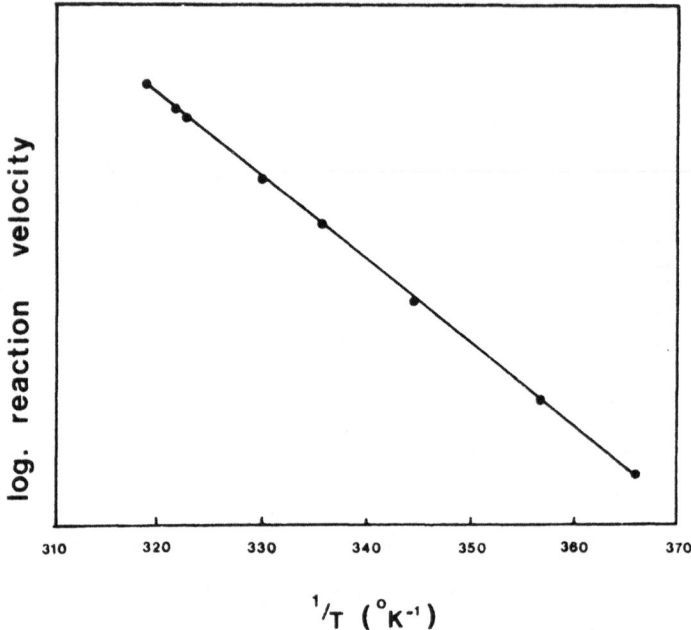

Fig. II.4. Arrhenius plot of the data in Fig. 3.

where T is absolute temperature, a and b are positive constants. Often the reaction velocity (v), which is a function of several different k's and substrate concentrations, will show a more complicated type of temperature dependency that also differs with other reaction conditions. For chromogenic substrates this relationship is demonstrated in Fig. II.4.

It is seen that in the range of room temperature a temperature rise of 1°C causes a rise in reaction velocity of between 2.5 and 7.5%. This demonstrates clearly the need for accurate temperature control.

This first of all holds within a series of experiments in one laboratory where velocities are to be compared within the series. However, when reaction velocities have to be compared between laboratories, temperature obviously is one of the variables that has to be rigorously standardized.

In experiments in which not only the splitting of the chromogenic substrate is involved but also one or more steps of the generation of the active enzyme, like thrombin generation, followed by the splitting of a chromogenic substrate, the latter may as well not be the reaction that governs the temperature dependence.

Coagulation reactions involve lipid – protein and protein – protein interactions. These may have very different numerical values for a and also a may change abruptly with temperature e.g. at the melting point of a lipid component (6). This prevents any general theoretical approach and makes accurate testing of the temperature behaviour of a system a necessity.

The temperature dependence of protein denaturation is usually much more pronounced than that of an esterolytic or amidolytic splitting. This is why enzyme solutions are best kept in the cold. A practical point arises here. If enzyme-containing solutions are to be added to a reaction mixture either the temperature of the reaction medium drops upon addition or the enzyme-solution has to be kept at the reaction temperature. In practice a compromise is sought. In precise biochemical experiments only small amounts of cooled enzyme solution are added to a reaction mixture of the right temperature. In routine clinical chemistry enzyme samples are usually kept at room temperature or near it. In enzymology the standard temperature is 25°C. In clinical chemistry one has as yet not decided firmly between 25°C, 30°C (room temperatures) or 37°C (body temperature).

Anyhow, whatever temperature is chosen, it is necessary to measure the reaction in a thermostated cuvette housing and to have a thermostate bath at hand to contain the stock solutions. As it is easier to heat cuvettes than to cool them, the standard temperature is best chosen above the ambient temperature.

II.5. The reaction medium

The activity of any enzyme will vary with pH and ionic strength and often is specifically influenced by certain ions. The medium in which an enzymatic reaction is measured has to be defined in these respects. When one specific enzyme has to be measured it is to be preferred to determine the optimal conditions and to apply these in the assay. As different enzymes often have different pH optima, the selectivity of an assay will be improved by measuring at the pH optimum of the enzyme to be determined. This is however not always the case. Plasmin e.g. has a narrow optimum at pH 7.4. At this pH urokinase also has near optimal activity. At pH 8.4, the plasmin is less active, whereas urokinase, that has a much broader pH optimum, still functions well. Urokinase activity therefore is preferentially measured slightly at the basic side of its pH optimum. Another reason to measure near the pH optimum is that small changes of pH around the optimal value will hardly bring about changes in enzyme activity.

It should be kept in mind that both K_m and k_{cat} are pH dependent and not necessarily both in the same way. Kinetic calculations therefore are only strictly valid with the constants obtained at that specific pH. The differences need not be large when the pH deviations are small.

The following working pH values are most often quoted. In brackets the ionic strengths most often used are indicated. Thrombin, 8.3 (0.15); factor X_a, 8.3 (0.25); plasmin, 7.4 (0.15); trypsin, 8.1 (0.15); papain 7.1 (0.15); brinase 7.6 (0.15); kallikrein, 7.9 (0.05); urokinase 8.4 (0.30).

The most common buffers are Tris/HCl and Tris/imidazole. Imidazole has been observed to inhibit trypsin and plasmin (P. Friberger, personal communication).

The ionic strength is obtained with NaCl. Apart from buffer and salts it may be necessary to add specific substances to the reaction medium: 0.1% Na-azide can prevent bacterial growth; 0.1%–0.5% carbowax 6000 (polyethyleneglycol, PEG) will prevent absorption of enzymes onto the walls of the cuvette. This is especially important when low concentrations of (purified) enzyme are used. With plasma samples and in general at relatively high protein concentrations this problem does not arise. Instead of carbowax, 1% ovalbumin or serum albumin can be used. In this case a check for the absence of activity in the albumin should be made.

Inhibitors

In some instances the specificity of a test can be improved by adding an inhibitor specific for unwanted activity e.g. hirudin for thrombin, or aprotinin for plasmin.

II.6. Substrate solution

In order to make an enzymatic reaction a suitable indicator of the amount of enzyme present, two conditions must be met.

a. The substrate should preferably be added at a concentration at least two times K_m, but
b. also the amount of colour produced should be easily measurable.

To meet the latter requirement, one should like to see $5 \mu M$ or more of product (absorbancy change 0.065 A) produced in the first 'linear' part of the reaction. We define the linear part of the reaction as that part in which no more than 5% drop of the initial velocity is observed.

A 5% drop of velocity due to substrate consumption is seen when more than 5% of substrate is consumed. So we remain on the safe side if we take $5 \mu M$ mentioned above as 5% of the initial substrate concentration. In other words, a substrate concentration of 0.1 mM will, if it is not much below $2 K_m$, be sufficient to suitably record the reaction. Circumstances do occur where K_m is greater than 2.10^{-4} M so 0.1 mM should be regarded as a minimal concentration but not as the optimal one.

It should be mentioned that contrary to general belief, it is not always necessary to measure initial velocities. It is indeed possible to measure the mean velocity over a certain time lapse but in that case the arithmetic mean substrate concentration over that time lapse should be used instead of the initial substrate concentration (7).

In this case substrate depletion up to a considerable amount will not hamper the validity of the Michaelis-Menten approach. Instead of formula 1.3, the formula becomes:

$$\frac{1}{\bar{v}} = \frac{1}{V} + \frac{K_m}{V}(1 + \alpha)\frac{1}{\bar{S}}$$

where $\bar{v}$ and $\bar{S}$ indicate the mean velocity and substrate concentration and α is a small positive value indicating the error introduced. α is below 0.01 when 30% of S is consumed and below 0.04 when the reaction is halfway to completion. The lowest velocity that can be measured with some accuracy in a current spectrophotometer is about 0.01 A/min (i.e. about $5\,\mu$M over 5 min). This $5\,\mu$M may represent as much as 50% of the initial substrate concentration. Even then, if the *mean* velocity over the time of observation is calculated and regarded as an initial velocity obtained at the *mean* concentration over that period the kinetic constants applicable will not show an error of more than 1%.

Example.
  Initial substrate concentration $10\,\mu$M
  After 5 minutes $4.6\,\mu$M has been consumed
  Mean reaction velocity $46/5 = 9.2\,\mu$M/min
  Mean substrate concentration $(10 + 5.4): 2\,\mu$M $= 7.7\,\mu$M
  These results therefore may be treated as if an initial reaction velocity of $9.2\,\mu$M was obtained at a substrate concentration of $7.7\,\mu$M.

K_m's for different enzyme-substrate complexes may vary from about $10^{-5} - 10^{-1}$ M. Some substrates are sparingly soluble in water (S 2160: 1.5 mM), and even less in the reaction medium. Relatively high amounts of substrate solutions therefore may have to be added to the reaction medium. In that case its influence on the pH and ionic strength should be taken into consideration.

The substrates are best solved in steril distilled water not above a temperature of 50°C. This will give a pH of 4−6. Maximal stability is obtained around pH 4. A small amount of acetic acid (2−5 mM) can be added to maintain the pH at 4. Lower pHs are to be avoided as they can cause acid hydrolysis of the`substrate. If substrate solution is added to the reaction mixture the final pH should be checked. The solutions are stable for at least 1 month at 5°C or below. No destruction by light has been observed. Probably all substrates can be kept for more than six months at room temperature if under sterile conditions. Microorganisms may break down the substrate rather quickly. Nitroaniline formation is in these cases seen as the first sign of breakdown. A drop of thymol added will guard against microbial growth.

II.7. Methodology

In a simple experiment three components have to be added together. The bulk consists of the reaction medium; enzyme and substrate are added separately afterwards. Conditions are chosen such that the concentration of the enzyme critically determines the rate whereas the substrate is present in excess. Therefore, precise pipetting of the enzyme is of the utmost importance, more important than that of the substrate solution.

As the enzyme solution mostly will be held on ice to avoid denaturation, the temperature will drop upon its addition. With modern automatic pipettes small volume can usually be added with great precision. A few minutes ($\frac{1}{2}$–2) after addition of the enzyme the reaction can be started by addition of the substrate previously brought to the right temperature. When only a small amount of enzyme is added to avoid an important drop in temperature, the reaction can as well be started in that way. This even is obligatory in two stage assays, where the generation or disappearance of the enzyme is monitored by subsampling from the primary reaction mixture into the reaction mixture containing the chromogenic substrate. Chromogenic substrates can also be used to monitor the appearance of an enzyme directly in the same mixture where the substrate is present. The thrombin generation in plasma after addition of thromboplastin and Ca^{2+} can e.g. be observed in this way. Here too, the reaction cannot be started by substrate.

The volume of the reaction mixture will be a compromise between the desired precision, that increases with the reaction volume and the cost of the reactants. This not only holds for the expensive chromogenic substrates, but especially in biochemical work also for the purified coagulation factors or other enzymes.

A large addition of enzyme solution will cause a considerable drop of temperature. A small quantity will be less accurately added than a large one. In practise again a compromise between these two effects will have to be sought.

II.8. Execution of the experiment

Conceptually the most simple setup is the addition of an amount of enzyme to the reaction medium containing chromogenic substrate after

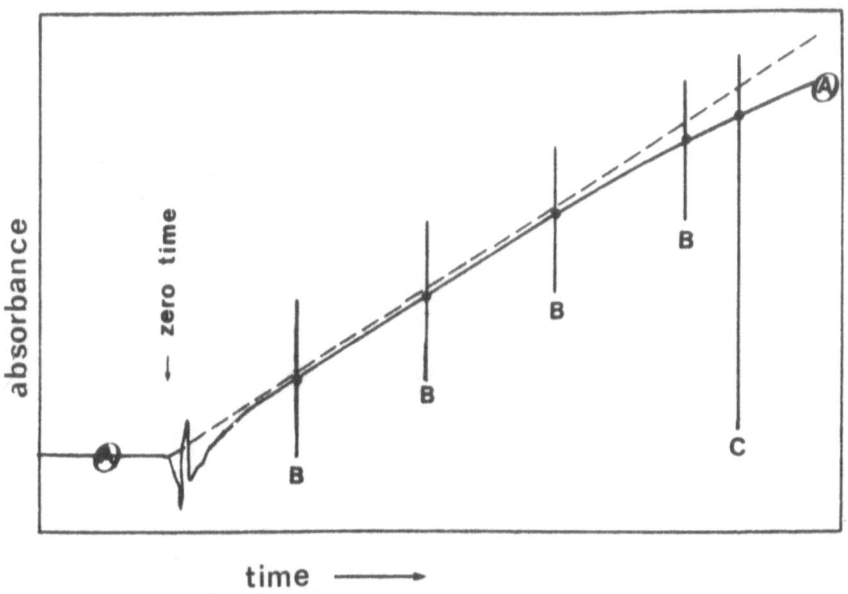

Fig. II.5. Time course of a simple reaction. Dotted line: ideal situation; drawn line: more realistic situation. A: continuous registration; B: Measuring points for an interval measurement; C: End point measurement.

which the change of optical density is registered graphically (Fig. II.5). In an uncomplicated reaction, the line obtained is straight if S is high enough and its slope indicates units of O.D. change per unit time, which, because the molar extinction of the product is known at the wavelength used, can directly be converted into a velocity of product formation (Fig. II.6). In this case graphic registration is hardly necessary except for control. The extinction can also be read at one or preferably more known intervals after zero time. As a third possibility the reaction can be stopped at a known time (end point method e.g. by adding 1/10 vol of 50% acetic acid).

Acids that will bring the pH considerably below 4 are to be avoided because of the risk of non-enzymatic acid hydrolysis of the substrate. Also the colour of *p*-nitroaniline disappears at low pH. The last method needs less equipment and is easily automated. Endpoint methods are especially useful when long reaction times are necessary and/or when many parallel measurements have to be carried out, because they need not be done in the spectrophotometer itself. It is absolutely necessary to make sure that the end point measured lies at straight part of the product-formation curve, however. After stopping the reaction with acetic acid, the colour is stable for at least four hours but care should be taken to prevent evaporation. End point methods only give a good

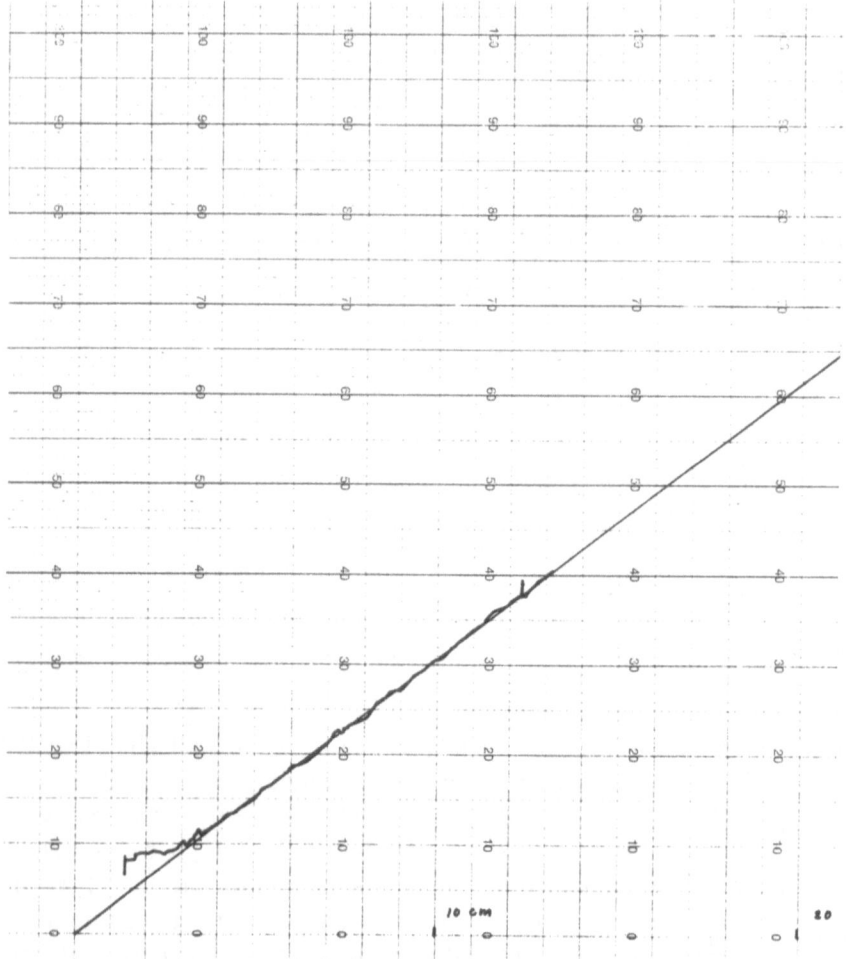

Fig. II.6. Calculation of reaction velocity from a strip chart recording. The slope of the curve is 61.5 divisions along the ordinate for 20 cm along the abscissa. Full scale is 100 divisions and corresponds to 0.50 optical density units. 61.5 divisions therefore correspond to $0.615 \times 0.50 = 0.308$ A. The paper speed was 2 cm/minute. The velocity of colour production therefore was 0.0308 A per min. As $\epsilon = 1.3 \times 10^4$ the velocity of the reaction was $3.08 \times 10^{-2} : 1.3 \times 10^4 = 2.4 \times 10^{-6}$ M per minute.

estimation of the initial reaction velocity if over the time interval used the rate does not rise or drop. In end point experiments usually a number of these tests is carried out simultaneously. In a parallel and comparable test no enzyme is added (blank). After a fixed incubation time (say 15 min) the reaction is stopped by adding acid. Then the O.D. of each of the solutions is read against the blank. When an O.D. of say 0.464 is measured, the O.D. before stopping the reaction was $11/10 \times 0.464 =$

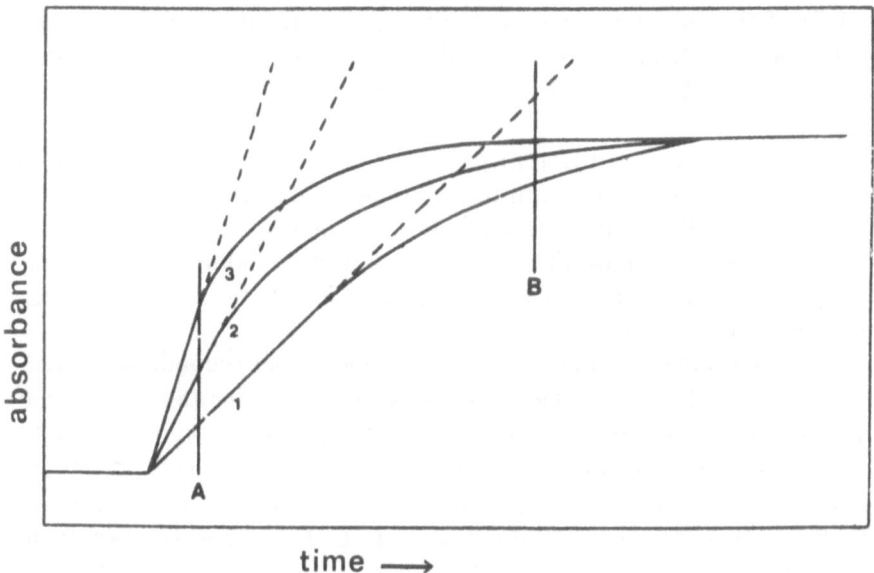

Fig. II.7. Time courses in a reaction where substrate is exhausted. 1, 2 and 3 indicate three reactions with enzyme concentrations in the proportions 1:2:3 and hence with initial velocities in these proportions. This proportion is found in an end point measurement if A is chosen as the end point but not at all if B is the endpoint.

0.510 A beacuse of the dilution by 1/10 vol 50% acetic acid. The rate of the reaction was 0.510/15 = 0.034 A per minute which corresponds to

$$0.034 : 1.3 \times 10^{-4} = 2.6 \times 10^{-6} \text{ M per min.}$$

When endpoint methods are applied it should be made sure that indeed the endpoint used under all circumstances lies on the straight part of the product-time graph. When appreciable lag times do occur or when the velocity drops, end point measurements are not accurate (Fig. II.7). Methods employing discontinuous readings do indicate such phenomena and therefore are applicable under these circumstances. End point measurements can be used even when they do not measure the reaction rate exactly. They then will be of the 'bio assay' type, for a discussion of which we refer to chapter IV.

The cause of the lag phases and declining velocities vary. Theoretically, a small lag phase always occurs because of the building up of the enzyme substrate complex. This, however, is in the millisecond range and does not have practical consequences. Mixing phenomena, temperature drop, recorder lag etc. may all contribute to an observed lag phase.

A decline in velocity can be due to a number of causes like exhaustion

(Fig. II.7) of the substrate or to instability or inactivation of the enzyme. Instability and inactivation have to be dealt with independently by finding conditions (pH, tube material, ionic strength etc.) under which they do not occur.

Product inhibition is a different case as it does not influence the initial reaction velocity. It would complicate things when mean velocities are used instead of initial velocities, as in the Lee and Wilson type of evaluation of experimental data. That method is only valid if product inhibition is absent. In practice, it is best to seek circumstances where these phenomena do not occur.

Reaction velocities are best expressed in moles per second. When K_m is known under the prevailing conditions, an experimentally measured velocity can be converted into katals: 1 katal being the amount of activity that converts 1 mol of substrate per second at infinite substrate concentration at defined (standard) conditions. A katal thus is a unit in which V_{max} is expressed. Its dimension is $C \cdot t^{-1}$. This follows from the relation:

$$v_{exp} = \frac{V \cdot S}{K_m + S} \quad \text{or} \quad V = k_{cat} E = v_{exp} \cdot \frac{K_m + S}{S}$$

When working at a known substrate concentration the term $(K_m + S)/S$ has a fixed value. When k_{cat} is known under the prevailing circumstances (dimension, t^{-1}) the enzyme concentration is easily calculated from the relation $V = k_{cat} \cdot E$. Using the katal is thus a step in obtaining E from v_{exp} via the Michaelis Menten relationship. Milli, micro and nano katals are defined as 10^{-3}, 10^{-6} and 10^{-9} katals, respectively.

An older convention uses the international unit of enzyme activity (IU) defined as the activity that splits 1 μmol substrate per minute:

1 IU = 1.67×10^{-8} mole/sec
1 mole/sec = 60×10^6 IU

When an enzymatic activity corresponding to 1 IU has to be expressed in katals, V_{max} must be obtained from v_{exp}, with the formula given above. This yields the following relationship:

$$1 \text{ IU} = 1.67 \times 10^{-8} \cdot (K_m + S)/S \text{ katals}$$

From this it will be clear that the expression of an enzymatic activity in katal units is appropriate only if the nature of the substrate and the reaction conditions are specified.

Measuring enzymatic activities as indicated above is relatively straightforward but it does not cover practice when working with coagulation enzymes. When e.g. to a medium containing a chromogenic substrate sensitive to thrombin, plasma, Ca^{2+} and thromboplastin are added,

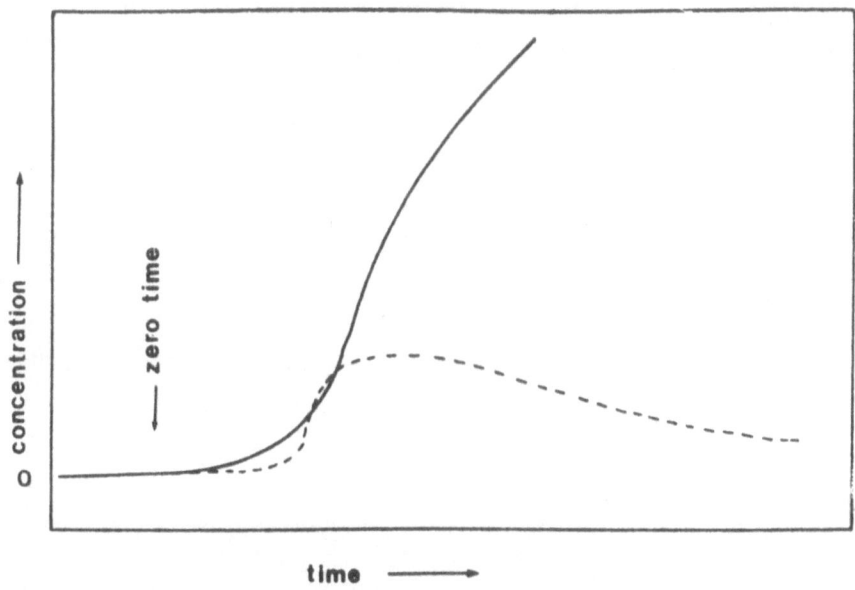

Fig. II.8. Thrombin generation. Thrombin generation (dotted line) and the ensuing conversion of S 2238 (drawn line) in a reaction mixture containing plasma, thromboplastin, Ca^{2+} and S 2238. Ca^{++} is added at zero time. (In practice S 2238 will cause a marked inhibition of prothrombinase!)

thrombin will generate and colour will develop. The time course of product formation, however, is very complicated (Fig. II.8).

When we assume the product formation to be proportional to the amount of thrombin present, the first derivative of the product formation curve will represent the thrombin concentration as a function of time. This curve itself is determined by the amount of prothrombin and the amounts of (potential) prothrombin activators present in the plasma added. Less plasma would cause a thrombin generation curve with both a longer lag time and a lower top activity but as there would be also less antithrombin III, the decrease of activity would also be slower (Fig. II.8).

It will be evident that such curves are hard to analyse. This type of situation is very often encountered in practice. It can be used for quantitative measurements by comparing samples to be tested to a series of dilutions of standard plasma (or other convenient preparations). When e.g. an end point measurement is carried out in the experiment illustrated in Fig. II.9 at the time indicated, the amount of colour found will depend in an unknown way on the amount of prothrombin (etc.) present in the sample. By comparing an unknown sample with a series of dilutions of a standard plasma it can be found out to what dilution of normal plasma

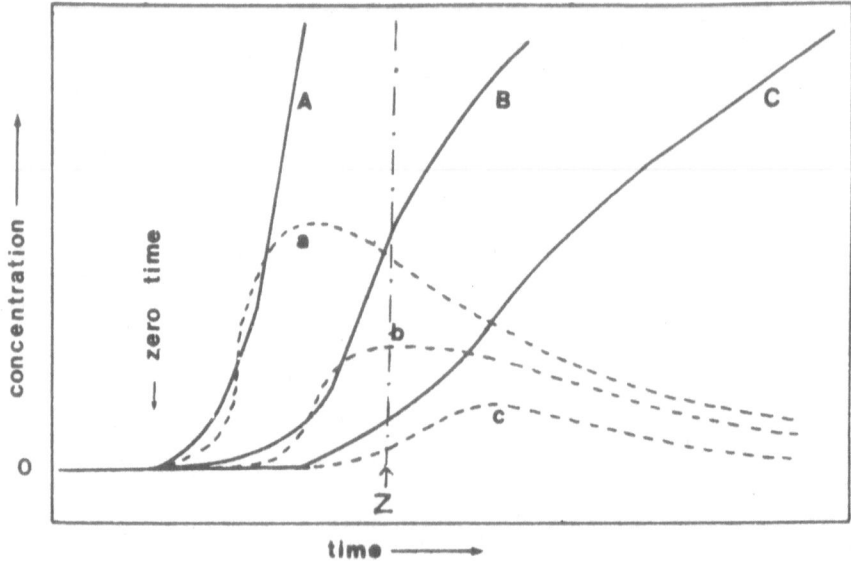

Fig. II.9. Thrombin generation. A, B and C indicate plasmas with decreasing thrombin generating potency. *Z* is an arbitrary point at which an end point determination is carried out (see text).

the sample corresponds. In essence this type of test, like the conventional clotting tests, is more like a pharmacological bioassay than like a biochemical rate measurement (see chapter IV).

Such bioassays are not necessarily more specific or more accurate than an assessment based on clotting time measurements. It does have more appeal to the chemical inclined, though.

II.9. Fluorescence

II.9a. General principles

Fluorescence is the phenomenon of the immediate emission of light by a molecule after the absorption of radiation. Under the circumstances we encounter in practice the wavelength of emission is always longer than that of the absorbed light. When studied in the range of visible and near ultraviolet light (200—800 nm) the phenomenon is due to electronic changes in the molecule. Fluorescence causes a sample irradiated by a beam of light to emit light in all directions. Two other phenomena have the same effect. Rayleigh scattering and Raman scattering. In Rayleigh scattering the light coming from the sample has the same wavelength as the incident beam. It occurs at all wavelengths but increases with the fourth power of the wavelength (hence the blue sky and the red setting sun). The Raman effect is related to Rayleigh scattering. It causes satellites with a higher wavelength then the Rayleigh peak; the constant wavelength difference from the exciting light that is characteristic of the molecular structure of the sample. Non fluorescent components of the sample (e.g. the solvent) do show scattering.

It is characteristic of fluorescence that it is caused by adsorption of light by a certain type of molecule. The excitation spectrum i.e. the wavelength that causes fluorescence is therefore identical to the adsorption spectrum of that molecular species. The fluorescent spectrum, the light emitted by the excited molecule is also characteristic for the species.

II.9b. Advantages and drawbacks

The advantages of fluorescence over spectrophotometry are twofold:

a. Specificity. Because two species characteristic wavelengths are necessary for measuring fluorescence, viz the excitation and the emission peak, this combination is apt to be more specific for one molecular species in a mixture than absorbancy that is measured at one wavelength only.

b. Sensitivity. Because the sample molecules act as the source of fluorescent light, no signal is observed when no sample molecules are present, and a small signal with low concentrations of sample. In photometric measurements the signal is maximal at zero concentration of the sample and low concentrations cause a small decrease of the maximal signal. It is understandable that the latter setup is essentially less sensitive.

The drawbacks of fluorescence are primarily the relative unfamiliarity of the technique and the fact that the apparatus is not generally available in all laboratories. Also the tricks of the method are not as well know to researchers and technicians etc. Before starting fluorimetry the reader is encouraged to read a text that more amply treats the matter than is possible in the context of this book (8).

Two important technical details are

1. The effect of scattering. Imperfect shielding and filtering of the incident beam can cause spurious signals. This is detected by using a non fluorescent but opalescent (i.e. strongly scattering) solution (like glucogen) as a sample.

2. The effect of temperature. As a rule fluorescence *decreases* when the temperature increases. The decrease occurring between 20°C and 30°C may be anything between 5 and 50% depending on the fluorescent

species and the solvent. Not only should the sample be always of the same temperature when put into the apparatus, but also the effect of heating by the incident light beam should be considered.

3. The effect of adsorption. In a sample even moderately adsorbing at the exciting wavelength, the energy of the incident beam decreases markedly with the length of path in the cuvette. Therefore at high concentration of the sample fluorescence will not increase lineary with concentration. In fact at very high concentrations it will decrease again. As a rule of thumb it may be assumed that fluorescence is linear with concentration as long as less than 5% of the incident energy is lost in the sample. I.e. as long as the adsorbancy of the sample is < 0.025. This also indicates that the concentration range in which fluorescence can be used is roughly one order of magnitude lower as that in which the same substance could be measured spectrophotometrically.

4. The effect of the reaction medium. Usually fluorescence is dependent upon the degree of ionisation of the substance to be measured, as the ionised and the unionised molecules have different fluorescence characteristics. Also the composition of the medium may influence the 'quantum yield' (see below) and thus influence the magnitude of the signal. Buffer composition therefore should be strictly controlled.

II.9c. Calculation of the results

Fluorescence increases with the intensity of the exciting light and, up to a certain limit with the concentration of the fluorescent species and the length of the optical light path. The intensity is emitted in all directions so only part of the energy emitted is sensed by the photomultiplyer.

The intensity of fluorescence is given by the following formula:

$$F = [P_0(1 - 10^{-\epsilon cb})][\phi] \qquad (2.6)$$

Where ϕ is the quantum yield. For the other symbols see Table II.3. If the amount of light adsorbed is small ($A < 0.025$) this equation can be simplified to

$$F = 2.3\, P_0\, \epsilon cb\, \phi \qquad (2.7)$$

from which it is clear that the amount of energy detected by the instrument is proportional to the concentration of the sample molecule.

The quantum yield (ϕ) is defined as the ratio of the number of light quanta emitted over the number absorbed. It can of course not be higher than unity. In aqueous solutions strongly fluorescent species like

Table II.3.   Symbols used in fluorescence

Symbol	Name
F	total fluorescence intensity (quanta per second)
P_0	intensity of exciting light (quanta per second)
c	concentration of the solution
b	optical depth of the solution
ϵ	molecular extinction coefficient
ϕ	quantum efficiency (yield) of fluorescence

fluoresceine and quinine have been reported to have quantum yields from 0.7 to 0.9 and from 0.3 to 0.6 respectively. This shows that the quantum yield is dependent upon the solvent i.e. upon buffer composition. Less strongly fluorescent molecules show proportionally lower quantum yields.

II.10. Electrochemical determinations (contributed by J.M. Nigretto)

II.10a. Principle of the method

Electrochemical determinations until now are in an experimental stage (9). They offer interesting and promising perspectives as they can be carried out in whole blood and in small volumes and are very sensitive.

The principle of the method is that not a chromophore is split off from an oligo-peptide but a residue that can be determined electrochemically, e.g. *p*-aminodiphenylamine (*p*ADA).

peptide–NH–⟨ ⟩–NH–⟨ ⟩ → peptide + NH₂–⟨ ⟩–NH–⟨ ⟩

for the different substrates possible see chapter III p. 89.

The concentration of the liberated diamine is determined periodically by measuring the current obtained by its electrochemical oxidation.

A scheme of the experimental setup is shown in Fig. II.10. It consists of the classical elements of electroanalysis.

- A signal generator, that with a velocity of ± 0.2 V/sec generates a triangular tension with an amplitude of -0.1 to 0.4 V against the calomel reference electrode. The signals can be produced continuously for the pretreatment of the electrode (see below) and at fixed intervals (automatically or by hand) during the actual measurement.
- A potentiostat that serves to maintain a constant instantaneous potential difference between the electrodes.
- The measuring cell in which the input (the changing potential between the electrodes) causes the response, i.e. the current between the working- and the counterelectrodes.

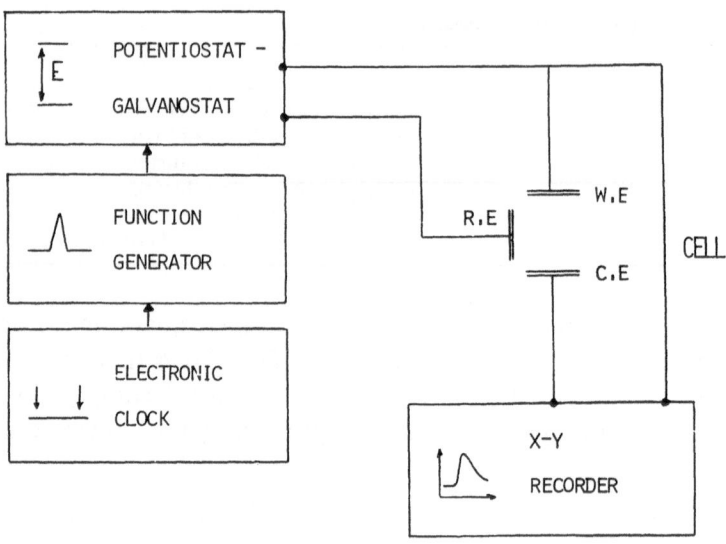

Fig. II.10. Scheme of the experimental set up for electrochemical determinations.

— The working electrode, consisting of a metal surface such as a platinum disk or metal vaporised in vacuum on a plastic support. Via this electrode the signal (voltage changes) is received and the resulting response (current changes) is measured.

— The counter electrode. A non corrosive metal thread suffices, if only the surface available is large compared to that of the working electrode in order to cause the electric current to flow through the circuit in which it is recorded, rather than through the reference electrode where the voltage is measured.

— The reference electrode, e.g. a saturated calomel electrode.

— The measuring cell is depicted in Fig. II.11. It is made of Teflon in order to minimise protein-surface interactions. The volume is 2 ml. It can be conveniently miniaturised to hold 0.5 ml without influencing the sensitivity of the method.

— Pretreatment of the working electrode is necessary because the interface current in a circuit with electrical electrodes is sensitive to the chemical state of this surfaces, especially to their oxidation. If the triangular signal is applied continuously for one minute in the solution in which the enzyme is to be measured before the enzyme is added, the electrode surfaces are in a reproducibly stable state and the same electrode can be used without need for regeneration during a series of measurements.

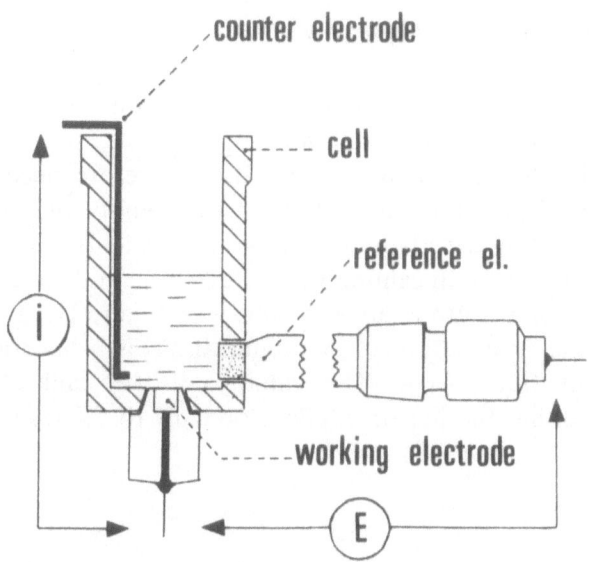

Fig. II.11. Measuring cell for electrochemical determinations.

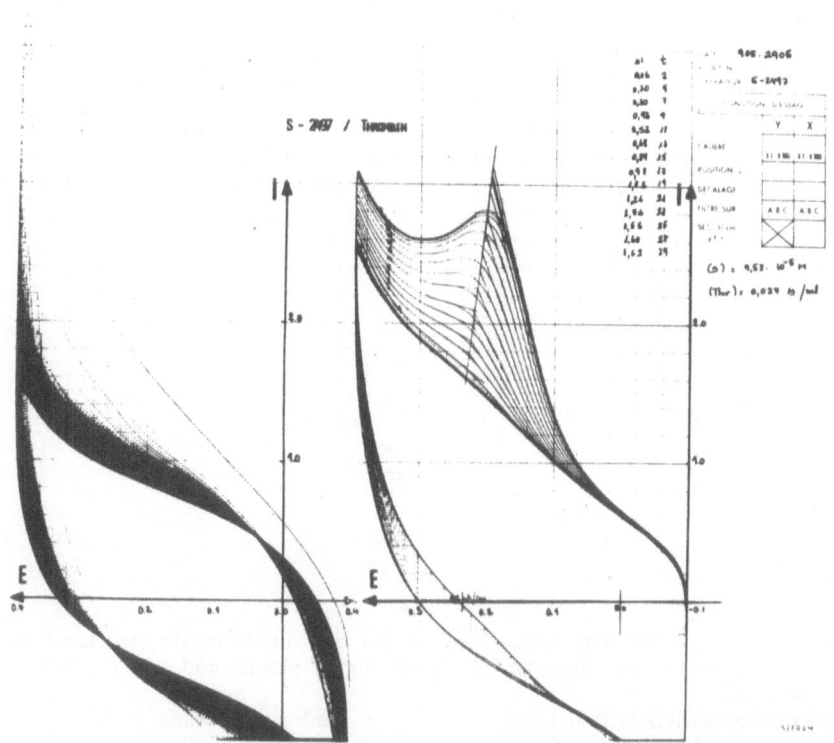

Fig. II.12. Series of curves obtained after the addition of 0.020 NIH U/ml of thrombin to 9.58×10^{-5} M of S2497 (H-D-Phe-pip-Arg-p ADA, 2 HCl).

II.10b. The determination of concentrations

The electrochemical signal is proportional to the concentration of *p*ADA but also dependent on the dimensions of the cell and electrodes, of the signal amplitude and frequency etc. It is therefore necessary that a calibration curve is established with known amounts of *p*ADA under the conditions of the test. Notably the volume and the buffer composition should be the same in calibration and experimental circumstances.

With each concentration a curve as shown in Figure II.12 is obtained. The heigth of the peak obtained at around 0.2 V is proportional to the concentration of free *p*ADA. The validity of the calibration is not influenced by adding plasma or whole blood up to 5% (*v/v*) of the cell

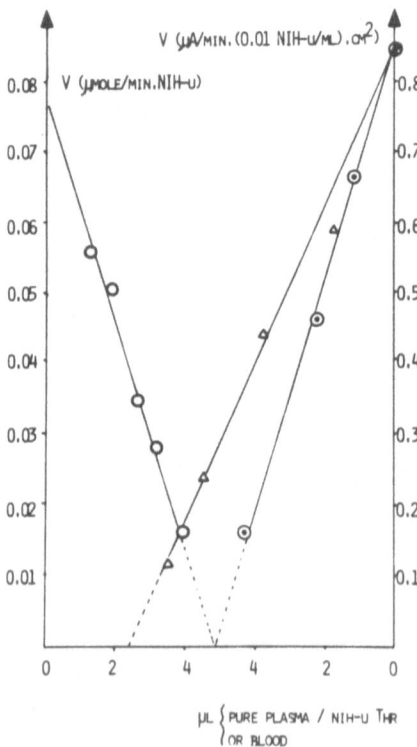

Fig. II.13. Electrochemical (right-hand scale) and photometric (left-hand scale) calibration curve of Antithrombin III from human plasma and whole blood (Thr. 0.4 NIH-U/ml)

Photometry with S-2238 0.1 mM	a — in human plasma
Electrochemistry with S-2497 0.1 mM.	b — in human plasma
c — in whole blood	c — in whole blood

Buffer: Tris/NaCl/Na₂ EDTA/Hep/DMSO pH 8.5, 37°C.

volume. At higher protein concentrations a different calibration curve made in the presence of (plasma) proteins is necessary.

Fig. II.12 shows a series of curves as obtained after the addition of 0.020 N.I.H.U/ml of thrombin to 9.58×10^{-5} M of S 2497 (H-D-Phe-pip-Arg-pADA, 2 HCl).

Fig. II.13 compares the results obtained in parallel electrochemical and spectrophotometrical determinations of antithrombin III.

References

1. Light and Living Matter. Vol. 1. The Physical Part. Clayton RK (ed). McGraw Hill Book Comp., New York, 1962
2. Experimental Techniques in Biochemistry. Brewer JM, Pesce AJ, Askworth RB (eds). Prentice-Hall Inc., New Jersey, 1974
3. The Tools of Biochemistry. Cooper TG. J. Wiley and Sons, New York, 1977
4. Instrumental Method of Chemical Analysis. 2nd ed. Ewing GW. McGraw Hill Book Comp., New York, 1969
5. Kaplan H, Laidler RJ: Can J Chemistry 45:547–552 (1969)
6. Tans G, Zutphen H v, Comfurius P, Hemker HC, Zwaal RFA: Eur J Biochem 95:225–233 (1979)
7. Lee HJ, Wilson IB: Biochim Biophys Acta 242:519–525 (1971)
8. Fluorescence Assay in Biology and Medicine. Udenfried S. Academic Press, New York, 1964
9. Daraio de Peuriot M, Nigretto JM, Jozefowicz M: Thromb Res 17:611–622 (1980)

III. Substrates

Summary

In this chapter the concepts of enzyme specificity and substrate selectivity
are introduced. The situation most often met in practice, i.e. that determinations have to be carried out in complicated biological systems with
not completely selective substrates, is discussed. Several approaches are
given to circumvent this lack of substrate selectivity. Also the inhibition
of the enzyme(s) to be tested by the artificial substrates and the consequences of this inhibition for the assays to be carried out are dealt with.

Finally the presently known artificial substrates are described. The
available data on chromogenic, fluorogenic, thioester, luminogenic substrates and substrates for electrochemical determinations are presented.

III.1. Specificity in serine proteases

Synthetic substrates are designed to assess quantitatively proteases that
have many properties in common. They have, therefore, to discriminate
between members of a family of very similar enzymes. The ideal chromogenic substrate is split at a considerable rate by one of these enzymes,
say thrombin, but is not split at all and is not even bound by a very
similar enzyme like factor X_a. In that case we define that it is *selective*
for thrombin. *Selectivity* is a property of the substrate, whereas *specificity*
is a property of the enzyme causing it to split certain substrates, but
not others. Selectivity and specificity are two sides of the same coin
because they are expressed only in the formation of the enzyme substrate
complex. In order to obtain insight in the possibilities and impossibilities
in this field a general discussion on substrate specificities of the serine
proteases is appropriate.

All serine proteases have the essentials of their catalytic mechanism
in common. They all split the same type of bonds: amides and esters
by the same series of chemical reactions. After the enzyme-substrate
complex has formed, the hydroxyl residue of the active serine engages

53

in a reaction with the substrate to form the tetrahedral complex (see also p. 12). The active serine is no. 195 in chymotrypsin (if not indicated otherwise, the numbering system in chrymotrypsin is used as a common reference). Serine 195 is so reactive because of its favourable juxtaposition to histidine 57 and other residues. By the interaction of the serine with the residues in its neighbourhood its nucleophilicity, and hence its reactivity is increased. The tetrahedral complex decomposes into the acyl enzyme and the leaving group (amine or alcolhol) of the substrate. In the acyl enzyme serine 195 is esterified with the carboxylgroup of the substrate. Esterification of serine 195 is a non-specific process that can in principle be carried out by any ester or amide that can obtain access to that serine. Evidently, the specificity of this group of enzymes is not to be found in the catalytic mechanism *per se*, but rather in the mutual accessibility of the active site and the vulnerable bond. Before an enzyme can split a substrate the two molecules have to bind first. With small substrates, this binding only concerns a small area at and near the active site. A proteolytic enzyme like factor X_a can split a small molecule like p-nitrophenylacetate, a larger molecule like S 2222, as well as a huge molecule like prothrombin. Between a small substrate and a large substrate, there will be hardly any difference as to the situation at the active site *per se*. In both cases, a similar type of bond is split. A large substrate, however, offers possibilities for contact with the enzyme over a much larger area than a small one. Over this area, various groups in the enzyme and the substrate have the possibility to interact and either attract or repulse each other. When the groups do attract, they will constitute an *accessory binding site* or *subsite*. It stands to reason that large molecules offer more possibilities for subsite interactions than small ones.

An increasing number of subsite interactions goes hand in hand with the possibility of a higher specificity just as an increasing number of indentations in a lock and key pair makes the combination safer. The high specificities of coagulation enzymes may depend on the fact that there are many subsite interactions. This implicates that there must be a theoretical limit to the selectivity of smaller substrates. Trypsin and chymotrypsin, on the other hand, being designed for general protein breakdown are inherently aspecific. For these enzymes subsite interactions are of less importance in the recognition of substrates. Any substrate that can be split by thrombin very probably will also be split by trypsin because at the active site the structural features are the same and subsites for trypsin hardly matter. Substrates selective for thrombin *only* therefore might be hard to find.

Before continuing the discussion on specificity it may be useful to try and define this concept in more detail. We can roughly discriminate between three types of specificity.

The first level concerns the type of chemical bond(s) involved. Serine proteases are specific for ester and amide bonds because of the mechanism outlined above; they will not attack double bonds or transfer electrons or close rings etc.

The second level of specificity is determined by the immediate vicinity of the bond under attack. Serine proteases have a 'pocket' in their surface near the active serine. The residue next to the esterifying carboxyl of the substrate has to fit snugly in this pocket in order for the acylation of the enzyme to proceed. Trypsin splits peptides and esters of the basic amino acids arginine and lysine, because its pocket is large enough to accommodate these residues and has a negatively charged aspartate residue at its bottom that forms a salt linkage with these positive groups. Chymotrypsin is specific for large hydrophobic side chains like phenylalanine, tyrosine and tryptophane. Elastase will split the bonds next to small hydrophobics like alanine. In summary: specificity of the first level is obtained by the chemical mechanism of enzymatic action per se: the making and disruption of covalent bonds. Specificity of the second level is obtained by the three-dimensional structure of the enzyme near the active serine.

The third level of specificity concerns the wider surroundings of the bond to be split. As an example, let us consider thrombin and trypsin acting on fibrinogen. In fibrinogen, there are scores of arginines many of which will be accessible from the outside so that in principle both enzymes should be able to reach them. Trypsin can indeed attack several of the arginine-bonds, but thrombin will only split off 2 times 2 fibrinopeptides per fibrinogen molecule. It therefore must be much more specific than trypsin. This may be caused by the fact that thrombin — possibly because of the presence of its A chain — will have more subsites available for positive interaction near the specific vulnerable sites of fibrinogen than trypsin has. On the other hand it has less possibilities for interaction near other potentially vulnerable (arginine or lysine) sites, because the same subsites that favour interaction in one place will counteract interaction in another. Indeed all coagulation proteases exhibit a very high specificity of the third level.

Modification of the thrombin molecule as can be caused by 'aging' or other, better defined modifications of the molecule will spoil some subsite interaction and render a thrombin that will not split fibrinogen but has an intact active centre, as can be judged from its patent esterase activity (1, 2). The same holds true for plasmin (3, 4). It should be kept in mind, though, that a large size of the enzyme and the substrate although it does create the possibility of enhanced specificity it does not guarantee it. The large enzyme plasmin e.g. will attack the large substrate casein in a rather random way like many other enzymes do.

All serine proteases of which the tertiary structure is known, appear to have a very similar spatial structure. The form of the 'backbone' of the molecule does hardly vary. Indeed much less than would be expected from the amount of identical or similar amino acids in the amino acid sequence (primary structure). This is because the amino acids at the inside of the molecule, that by their interactions are the main determinant for the form of the molecule, are conserved to a high extent (about 60%) during evolution. The amino acids that find themselves at the surface are quite variable and show only 10% of conserved sites. One could say that the different serine proteases have all more or less the same form but that the residues sticking out tend to be different. These residues can potentially interact with neighbouring molecules by weak chemical forces like v.d. Waals interaction and H-binding or by electrostatic interaction. A specific pattern of residues will therefore cause a specific mozaic of potential chemical interactions in space. If such a mosaic on the surface of a protease meets a complementary pattern on another protein, binding will be probable. When two proteins do not possess a complementary surface pattern in the region where they touch, the tendency to bind to each other will be small.

This type of interaction has been demonstrated for soybean trypsin inhibitor (SBTI) binding to trypsin. SBTI acts as a natural polypeptide substrate that does bind to the active site and subsites of trypsin (5). Unlike a substrate it will not dissociate. This results in a permanently occupied enzyme molecule. Therefore (SBTI) acts as an inhibitor. The SBTI-trypsin complex can be crystallized and its tertiary structure determined. It shows that the inhibitor and the enzyme touch and bind over a relatively large area as would be expected from the high specificity of the interaction.

This situation explains why chromogenic substrates can be relatively selective: if they mimic a natural substrate of a certain enzyme in that they are complementary to the surface mosaic of that enzyme they will be preferably bound. If they contain the right vulnerable site they will be split subsequently. Because they are much smaller than the natural substrate they will bind to fewer subsites than the normal substrate, and hence the binding will be less specific. Chromogenic substrates therefore are not likely to attain the degree of specificity of a natural substrate. It will be clear that to some extent knowledge of the primary structure of the natural substrate near its vulnerable site(s) may be useful. This is undoubtedly so for specificity of the second level. It is less evident for specificity of the third level because amino acids very near the vulnerable site in the sequence of the amino acids may lie at the inside of the enzyme molecule and play no role in the recognition between enzyme and substrate, whereas amino acids distant in the primary structure may lie at the surface quite near the active site. Therefore, the ideal chromogenic substrate cannot be designed on basis of knowledge of the primary structure of its natural substrate alone and there is a marked place for trial and error in finding it.

It was found e.g. that Ile-Glu-Gly-Arg is a common sequence preceding the bond specificity split by factor X_a and indeed Bz-Ile-Glu-Gly-Arg-pNA (S 2222) is a good substrate specifically for this factor (6). Upon the assumption of an α-helical structure of fibrinopeptide, it could be calculated that a *Phe*-residue would be in a position relative to the C-terminal Arg as also could be obtained by interposing only one amino acid (Val) in a linear structure. Indeed Bz-Phe-Val-Arg-pNA is a good substrate for thrombin (7, 8). On the other hand, no substrates for factor IX_a have as yet been found although the primary structure of factor X_a around its splitting site has been taken as a guideline (9, 10, 11).

III.2. Substrate selectivity and sensitivity

The common specificity of many plasma proteases for peptide bonds at the carboxyl side of basic amino acids (most frequently arginine) creates a very significant challenge if concentrations of individual proteases in a mixture are to be assayed independently. A completely specific enzyme would split only *one* substrate. However, enzyme *specificity* is usually limited, hence one enzyme may split various substrates, be it at different rates. Consequently, a given substrate can be split by various different enzymes present simultaneously in a given solution. The *selectivity* of the substrate determines by what enzyme it is preferably split. Specificity thus is a property of an enzyme. High specificity indicates that an enzyme has a strong or even exclusive preference for one substrate. Selectivity is a property of a substrate, high selectivity indicating that it is preferably − or even exclusively − split by one enzyme. S 2302 e.g. is not very selective although it has a preference for plasma kallikrein whereas S 2444 is highly selective for trypsin. Selectivity of the original substituted arginine chromogenic substrates has been increased by synthesis of oligopeptides of varying structure, but absolute selectivity has not been achieved in spite of many clever structural modifications in their constituent amino acid. An examination of the amino acid sequence specificity of plasma proteases such as thrombin and plasmin which can cleave several argininyl peptide bonds in different protein substrates, suggests that absolute specificity should not be expected.

As is explained on p. 24, selectivity is also a function of substrate concentration. Therefore, tables giving relative velocities at one substrate concentration are only of very limited use. The best parameter for selectivity is k_{cat}/K_m (see p. 6).

Sensitivity is related directly to the amount of coloured product that can be produced by unit amount of enzyme. When high enough substrate concentrations can be used, sensitivity is dependent upon k_{cat}. Sensitivity and selectivity are therefore basically unrelated.

From the situation described above it will be clear that one cannot expect to obtain highly selective substrates suitable for the independent assessment of the concentrations of one or several proteases in a complex mixture. Additional and alternative methods have to be found. Several approaches that increase the selectivity of protease assays exist and can alone, or in combination, be used for the assay of a given protease in the presence of other proteases of similar structure and overlapping specificity. It is indeed quite possible to do useful work with not completely selective substrates The approaches that make possible the independent estimation of the concentrations of each of several protease in a mixture are the following:

a. Work in a pure or otherwise well defined reaction mixture

If one wants to estimate thrombin generation by prothrombinase made from pure factor X, factor V_a and phospholipid by subsampling from the reaction mixture into a mixture containing chromogenic substrate, the only condition to be fulfilled in practice is that the substrate is not much more sensitive for factor X_a than for thrombin (12). It therefore can be aselective. In plasmas or other mixtures containing a host of potentially active enzymes, higher demands are made on the selectivity of the substrate, or the test system has to be designed so as to circumvent the complications that may arise.

b. Use of specific inhibitors

Several inhibitors exist that are more or less specific for given proteolytic enzymes. The inhibition may be either reversible or irreversible. Selective inhibition of particular proteases by irreversible inhibitors such as some of the protein protease inhibitors available from both plant and animal tissues, irreversible inhibitors prepared by chemical synthesis such as the peptide chloromethylketones (13) and peptide argininaldehydes (14), as well as reversible inhibitors prepared by chemical synthesis (15, 16, 17, 18) have all been exploited. Several of these inhibitors seem to be extremely specific, although many combinations of protease and inhibitor have not been investigated to date. Data available from the study of the inhibition of several proteases by the peptidylarginine chloromethyl-ketones (13) however suggest that absolute specificity will not exist with these inhibitors. This is not surprising because the affinity of an enzyme for these relatively small substances will be subject to the same limitations as that for the chromogenic substrates themselves.

Diisopropylfluorophosphate (DFP) and in general active site titrants inhibit irreveribly by covalent binding to the active serine. They can be useful because sometimes the affinity for one enzyme is much higher than for another. DFP e.g. will bind to and inhibit thrombin but hardly affect factor X_a. Other irreversible inhibitors are the natural inhibitors like soy bean trypsin inhibitor (SBTI), lima bean trypsin inhibitor (LBTI) or hirudin (see also p. 36) these are high molecular weight polypeptides and therefore can be highly specific. Substrates of any kind in principle act as competitive reversible inhibitors, because they occupy active sites. Tosyl arginine methyl ester (TAMe) will inhibit thrombin action on fibrinogen, because it is split by thrombin. Such substances are not very useful as inhibitors because

a. inhibition decreases in time with consumption of the inhibitor;
b. infinite concentrations of inhibitor are necessary to obtain complete inhibition.

 With pseudo-substrates that have a high binding constant but a low or absent rate of conversion (k_{cat}) the first objection does not count, but the second objection remains, although it may be quanti-tatively unimportant. Also non-competitive reversible inhibitors exist. ϵ-amino caproic acid inhibits plasmin in a complex way in the first place by binding to adjacent binding sites and only at high concen-trations by binding to the active site. Aprotinin (Trasylol®) is a poly-peptide that irreversibly inhibits plasmin etc. More examples of the use of inhibitors can be found in descriptions of individual assay systems.

c. *Kinetic analysis of the situation* (contributed by C. Jackson)

An approach which is capable of permitting estimation of the concen-trations of several proteases in a solution provided they are not identical in their kinetic parameters for the hydrolysis of chromogenic and fluoro-genic substrates exists and may be readily applied by anyone performing single substrate assays (19). This approach requires only that assays be carried out using either more than one substrate or at different concentrations of the same substrate and knowledge of the kinetic parameters which describe the hydrolysis of each of the substrates by the isolated, chemically homogeneous enzymes. The rapid progress in developing procedures for the isolation of essentially all of the known plasma proteases makes knowing the kinetic parameters possible and thus this approach to estimation of the amounts of individual proteases in a mixture attainable in the near future. The bases for this approach are set out below.

In a mixture of several enzymes each of which can act on the assay substrate the chromogenic product being formed results from the combined action of all the enzymes on the substrate. If initial velocities are measured from the reaction progress curve, then the measured velocity will be equal to the sum of the initial velocities of the reactions being catalyzed by each enzyme. This is most clearly expressed by the algebraic equation below where V_{tot} is the total velocity and $V_1 \ldots V_n$ are the velocity contributions of each enzyme which is present.

$$V_{(tot)} = V_{(1)} + V_{(2)} + V_{(3)} \tag{1}$$

From the relationship between initial reaction velocity and substrate concentration, which is given by the Michaelis-Menten equation, it can be deduced that at any given substrate concentration the reaction velocity contributed by each enzyme is equal to a constant for that enzyme times its concentration. The constant is characteristic for each enzyme, substrate and particular substrate concentration of that substrate. The total velocity can then be easily expressed as follows.

$$V_{(tot)} = C(1) \cdot E(1) + C(2) \cdot E(2) + \ldots + C(n) \cdot E(n) \tag{2}$$

The value of the constant for each enzyme is simply the following.

$$C(i) = k_{cat}(i) \cdot S/(K_m(i) + S) \tag{3}$$

Thus if the kinetic parameters for the hydrolysis of each substrate by the various enzymes are known, the proportionality constants can be calculated for any enzyme that is known to be present in the mixture.* In order to maximize the contribution of the enzyme of interest, it is desirable to use a substrate concentration or a 'specific' substrate whose selectivity for that enzyme maximizes its proportionality constant. The 'disadvantage' of this approach is only that as many different total velocity measurements with either different substrates or at different

---

*Extension of this approach to identification of which enzymes are most probably present is similarly possible, but its discussion is beyond the scope of this presentation.

substrate concentrations as there are enzymes must be made in order to determine the enzyme concentrations. The maximum number of proteases measurable with a given degree of accuracy remains to be established. If use is made of the current technology of clinical chemistry laboratories, this 'disadvantage' does not actually exist. The maximum of proteases measurable with a given degree of accuracy remains to be established. If independent evidence exists that indicates that some enzymes are present in very low concentration, these may be ignored with introduction of only minimal error. The issue of particular estimates is addressed below.

Calculation of the proportionality constants for each enzyme requires that values for the kinetic parameters, k_{cat} and K_m be known. These must be determined from measurements of reaction velocity as a function of substrate concentration for each of the enzymes and each of the substrates. When such data are available, specific design of assays for any particular plasma protease can be carried out. Although insufficient data currently exist to do this completely, ongoing efforts in several laboratories will make this possible in the future. However, even in the absence of complete data, the power of this approach can be illustrated by performing calculations for hypothetical values for k_{cat} and K_m and enzyme concentration. Table III.1(A) shows such illustrative calculations for a system of one substrate in which the K_m's for two different enzymes differ by a factor of 10 but k_{cat} is the same.

Table III.1.   Relative contributions of each of two proteases to the initial velocity of a reaction which they both catalyze.**

A. $K_m E_1 = 1.0\,\mu M$, $K_m E_2 = 10.0\,\mu M$, $k_{cat} = 10\,\mathrm{sec}^{-1}$ for each.

Relative contribution of enzyme (1)

Substrate (μM)	$E_1/E_2 = 10$	$E_1/E_2 = 1$	$E_1/E_2 = 0.1$
1.0	0.98	0.85	0.35
10.0	0.95	0.65	0.15
100.0	0.92	0.52	0.10

B. $K_m E_1 = K_m E_2$, $k_{cat} E_1 = 10\,\mathrm{sec}^{-1}$, $k_{cat} E_2 = 1\,\mathrm{sec}^{-1}$

1.0	0.99	0.91	0.50
100.0	0.99	0.91	0.50

**This is calculated as follows: $V(tot) = V(1) + V(2)$ i.e. $V(tot) = k_{cat}(1) \cdot E(1) \times S/(K_m(1) + S) + k_{cat}(2) \cdot E(2) \times S/(K_m(2) + S)$, and the relative contribution of $E(1)$ is equal to $V(1)/V(tot)$.

These calculations illustrate clearly that for enzymes which differ in K_m, selectivity in assay may be enhanced by choice of substrate concentration, but when only k_{cat} is different, substrate concentration is without effect on the relative contribution to the measured total reaction velocity. The best situation is when both K_m and k_{cat} favor the enzyme of interest, that is when k_{cat}/K_m is large. The benefit of having differences in K_m is that a single substrate may be used at different concentrations. However, this advantage may be offset by the increased difficulty in obtaining accurate estimates of the initial rate under these conditions because of the low substrate concentrations required to achieve the selectivity. This, however, depends on the actual values of the Michaelis constants (K_m's) for the particular enzymes. If only the k_{cat} values differ, then estimation of the concentration of a single protease in a mixture requires the use of different substrates and no gain in selectivity is obtained by altering the substrate concentration. However, in this case the substrate concentration may be chosen to provide the desired accuracy in initial velocity estimation or on the basis of cost of reagents, substrates, etc.

Calculation of the value of the coefficient for one term in equation (3) is illustrated in Table III.2. The calculation of enzyme concentration from knowledge of the coefficients for thrombin and Factor Xa acting on Tos-Gly-L-Pro-L-Arg-pNA (Chromozym TH) and Bz-L-Ile-L-Glu-Gly-L-Arg-pNA (S-2222) is illustrated in Table III.3.

Table III.2. Illustrative calculation of the coefficients for relating reaction velocity to enzyme concentration at fixed substrate concentration.

Chromozym TH	S-2222
Thrombin: $K_m = 3.6\,\mu M$, $k_{cat} = 102\,sec^{-1}$	$K_m = 55.6\,\mu M$, $k_{cat} = 0.94\,sec^{-1}$
Factor *Xa*: $K_m = 121\,\mu M$, $k_{cat} = 77.5\,sec^{-1}$	$K_m = 180.\,\mu M$, $k_{cat} = 149.\,sec^{-1}$

If the substrate concentration is $100\,\mu M$ in all cases, then:

$$C_{(\text{Thrombin on Chromozym TH})} = (102\,sec^{-1} \times 100\,\mu M)/(3.6\,\mu M + 100\,\mu M)$$

$$C_{(\text{Thrombin on Chromozym TH})} = 98.4\,sec^{-1}$$

Similarly, the coefficients for Factor Xa acting on $100\,\mu M$ Chromozym TH or S-2222 and thrombin on $100\,\mu M$ S-2222 can be calculated and are:

$$C_{(\text{Factor Xa on Chromozym TH})} = 35.1\,sec^{-1}$$

$$C_{(\text{Thrombin on S-2222})} = 0.604\,sec^{-1}$$

$$C_{(\text{Factor Xa on S-2222})} = 53.2\,sec^{-1}$$

Table III.3. Calculation of the concentrations of thrombin and Factor Xa in a mixture from measurement of the initial velocity of hydrolysis of Chromozym TH and S-2222.

If the initial velocity measured for a mixture of thrombin and Factor Xa acting on Chromozym TH is 0.163 abs/min (at 405 nm) and acting on S-2222 is 0.159 abs/min (at 405 nm) then the concentration of each enzyme is calculated as follows: (After converting absorbance/min to concentration/sec using a molar extinction coefficient for p-nitroaniline at 405 nm of $9920 \, M^{-1} \, cm^{-1}$.)

$$V(M \, sec^{-1}) = (Abs \, min^{-1} \, cm^{-1})/(9920 \, M^{-1} \, cm^{-1} \times 60 \, sec \, min^{-1}) \quad (4)$$

From the coefficients of Table III.1 and equation (2) for each of the two separate total velocity measurements:

$$V_{(Chromozym \, TH)} = 98.4 \, [thrombin] + 35.1 \, [Factor \, Xa] \quad (5)$$

$$V_{(S-2222)} = 0.604 \, [thrombin] + 53.2 \, [Factor \, Xa] \quad (6)$$

Subtracting 98.4 [thrombin] from $V_{(Chomozym \, TH)}$ in equation (5) and dividing by 35.1, the coefficient for Factor Xa gives:

$$[Factor \, Xa] = (0.274 \, \mu M \, sec^{-1} - 98.4 \, [thrombin])/35.1 \quad (7)$$

When this is substituted into equation (6) the concentration of thrombin is calculated to be 1 nM. The concentration of Factor Xa, 5 nm, is calculated from either equation (5) or (6).

Note: if the thrombin concentration is now substituted into the equation describing the initial velocity observed using S-2222 it can be seen that the contribution of thrombin is negligible to this reaction at this thrombin concentration.

This approach can be extended to several velocity measurements with some substrates and, thus, assay of many proteases in a mixture is possible. The accuracy with which each enzyme can be determined depends upon the selectivity of the substrates chosen for the assays and the accuracy with which the initial velocities of the reactions are measured. The solution of the simultaneous equations which arise from such multiple measurements can be awkward to obtain if the substitution method used above is employed. However, many small pocket calculators of the scientific variety incorporate ready-made programs for solving such sets of simultaneous equations. Until sufficient data are available to provide estimates for the accuracy of the reaction initial velocity measurements, assessment of the accuracy which can be achieved cannot be made.

Another method for increasing the selectivity of a reaction for any particular protease is to use a relatively specific competitive inhibitor of the other protease in the reaction mixture. Inclusion of such a competitive inhibitor alters the apparent K_m for each enzyme that it inhibits, (K_m apparent becomes equal to $K_m(1 + [INH]/K_i)$, but when the alteration is greater for the interfering ezymes than for the enzyme of interest, the effect is the same as increasing the difference in the K_m's for a particular substrate as illustrated in Table III.1(A) above. The total reaction velocity will also be reduced, but this requires only that a longer reaction time be employed for the measurement of the initial velocity. Obviously this approach requires knowledge of the inhibition constants, (K_i's) for the particular inhibitor and the relevant enzymes, but a considerable body of data for amidino compounds has already been obtained in the laboratories of Geratz (15), Markwardt (16, 17) and Okamoto (18).

Even though implementation of the approaches described above is currently limited by the unavailability of kinetic constants for the various enzymes and substrates, this situation is rapidly changing and thus implementation of this approach in the future will undoubtedly occur.

III.3. Inhibition by artificial substrates

An interesting situation can arise when an artificial substrate is added to a mixture where two enzymes are present and it binds to both, but is split mainly by one. Imagine that the substrate S is added to a mixture of factor X_a and prothrombin. In separate experiments, it has been shown that factor X_a hardly or not splits the substrate but that thrombin does. Can it then be safely assumed that the appearance of the product monitors the concentration of thrombin as if the chromogenic substrate were not present? The answer is no. It is quite possible that the chromogenic substrate binds to factor X_a and thereby acts as a competitive inhibitor of prothrombin conversion. In fact, if k_{cat} of factor X_a acting on the substrate is small, while K_m is in the order of magnitude of the substrate concentration, the K_m of the substrate for factor X_a will be the K_i of that substrate acting as an inhibitor of prothrombin conversion by factor X_a hence the velocity of prothrombin conversion (v) will be

$$v = \frac{k_{cat} \cdot [X_a] \, [II]}{[II] + K_{mp} \, (1 + S/K_{ms})}$$

where

$$[II] = \text{prothrombin concentration}$$
$$[X_a] = \text{factor } X_a \text{ concentration}$$
$$S = \text{concentration of chromogenic substrate}$$
$$K_{mp} = \text{Michaelis constant for prothrombin}$$
$$K_{ms} = \text{Michaelis constant for artificial substrate}$$
$$k_{cat} = \text{catalytic constant for prothrombin}$$

The k_{cat} for the action of factor X_a on the substrate does not figure in this formula. It can be so small that factor X_a is not considered to act on the substrate in question at all. This again illustrates how important it is to know the kinetic constants not only of the artificial substrates but also of the natural substrates.

In practise as has been shown by Orthner *et al.* (21) the inhibition exercised by small molecular weight substrates is not purely competitive but may be of a mixed type.

Mutual competitive inhibition obviously makes the approach to test several enzymes in the presence of several substrates as outlined in III.2. still possible but more difficult in practise. If however the inhibitions are of a mixed type not only the K_m 's but also all the mutual K_i's would be necessary for the calculations and practical applicability would soon approach zero.

III.4. Data on commercially available substrates

In the following part the chemical and kinetic data of the most common commercially available substrates are given. Again it should be stressed that the values of the kinetic constants are only rough indications not meant to be used for anything else but for approximate calculations of substrate concentrations required or the order of magnitude of reaction velocities to be expected. In fact the dependence of K_m and k_{cat} on reaction circumstances (pH, ionic strength, concentrations of non-enzyme proteins, concentration of specific ions etc.) makes it obligatory to determine K_m in every individual experimental setup if it is necessary to have an exact knowledge of this constant. More precise data applicable under specified conditions are to be found in the literature. We decided not to use these as it would be impossible to include all relevant reaction circumstances, so that the reader would have to consult the original publications anyhow.

Detailed information on kinetic parameters of isolated factors in a medium consisting of 0.01 M HEPES, 0.01 M Tris/HCl pH 7.8, 0.1 M NaCl and 0.1% polyethyleneglycol 6000, not containing other proteins *or* 0.05 M Tris/HCl, 0.1 M NaCl, pH 8 also in absence of other proteins, are to be found in ref. (22).

Table III.4. List of the main commercially available *p*-Nitroaniline containing substrates.

No	shorthand chemical name	commercial name	Mol. weight	substrate for:
1	b-ile-glu-gly-arg-pNA	S 2222	741.3	factor X_a
2	b-ile-glu-pip-gly-arg-pNA	S 2337	801.5	factor X_a
3	pglu-gly-arg-pNA	S 2444	498.9	urokinase
4	b-val-gly-arg-pNA	Chromozym UK	599.1	urokinase
5	D-val-leu-arg-pNA	S 2266	579.6	gland. kallikrein
6	b-pro-phe-arg-pNA	Chromozym PK	679.3	plasma kallikrein
7	D-pro-phe-arg-pNA	S 2302	611.6	plasma kallikrein
8	D-phe-pip-arg-pNA	S 2238	635.6	thrombin
9	t-gly-pro-arg-pNA	Chromozym TH	639.1	thrombin
10	D-ile-pro-arg-pNA	S 2288	577.6	thrombin and others
11	b-phe-val-arg-pNA	S 2160	681.2	thrombin and others
12	D-val-leu-lys-pNA	S 2251	551.5	plasmin
13	t-gly-pro-lys-pNA	Chromozym PL	611.1	plasmin
14	cmprop-arg-pro-tyr-pNA	S 2586	705.3	chympotrypsin
15	pglu-pro-val-pNA	S 2484	445.5	g. elastase

Meaning of the abbreviations (alphabetical).

arg	ariginine	phe	phenylalanyl
b	N-benzoyl	pip	γ-piperidyl
cmprop	carbomethoxypropionyl	pNA	para nitro anilide
D	dextro configuration*	pro	propyl
glu	glutamyl	pyl	pipecolyl
gly	glycyl	t	N-tosyl
ile	isoleucyl	val	valyl or valine
leu	leucyl		
lys	lysine		*If no D is written the laevorotary forms
pglu	pyroglutamyl		of the aminoacids are meant.

1. b-ile-glu-gly-arg-pNA · HCl

substrate for: factor X_a
commercial name: S 2222

Chemical name:	N-Benzoyl-L-isoleucyl-L-glutamyl-glycyl-L-arginine-p-nitroanilide hydrochloride and its methyl ester

Formula:

in half of the material R=H, in half R=CH$_3$

Mol. weight:	734.3 (R=H) and 748.3 (R=CH$_3$) 741.3 can be used in practise.
E_{max}:	1.28×10^4 mol^{-1}. l. cm^{-1} (λ_{max}: 316 nm in water)
Solubility:	6 mmol. l^{-1} in H$_2$O 2 mmol. l^{-1} in Tris buffer (pH 8.3, I 0.25)
Stability:	Dry substance stable at room temperature Slightly hygroscopic Solution (4 mM/l in water) stable for more than 6 months at room temperature. Contamination by microorganisms may cause hydrolysis.

Stock solution
As the K_m for factor X_a is relatively high (see below) it is important to obtain exactly identical starting concentrations of this substrate if reproducible results are to be obtained. This is best done by solving the contents of one vial (á 25 mg) in 7.5 ml of solvent so as to obtain a solution of about 4.4 mM. Estimation of O.D. 316 of a 1:100 dilution will yield a figure of above 0.500 O.D.U. (say 0.560). Then the stock solution is diluted so as to make the optical density of the solution equal to 50. (In our example by adding (6/50) × 7.5 ml to the stock solution.) The concentration of the stock solution then will be 3.90 mM. If this is diluted 1:20 in a test a final concentration of 195 μM is reached.

Data
The K_m of factor X_a acting on this substrate is around 300 μM (pH 8.2, Tris buffer, I 0.25, 37°C); k_{cat} is around 100 sec^{-1}. Of course the values differ widely depending upon pH, I, temperature, other proteins present etc. and upon the type of factor X_a present (species, molecular variants).

For trypsin K_m is around $10\,\mu$M and k_{cat} approx. $300\,sec^{-1}$. The substrate is also readily split by subtilisin. Both these enzymes are not common contaminants of factor X_a reaction mixtures and hence need not disturb clotting factor estimations. Under the conditions mentioned above for the estimation of factor X_a, thrombin will split the substrate at $< 3\%$ of the rate obtained with factor X_a. As the potential concentration of thrombin in plasma mixtures is up to $10 \times$ that of factor X_a, thrombin is a contaminant to be reckoned with. Hirudin may be used as a specific thrombin inhibitor or the fact that factor X_a is relatively insensitive to the inhibitory action of diisopropyl-fluorophosphate (DFP) may be made use of. Plasma kallikrein if fully activated in a plasma mixture could contribute to hydrolysis to up to 15% of the potential activity of factor X_a. Plasmin even up to 25%. Prevention of cold activation and activation of the fibinolysis system (EACA, Trasylol) may therefore be advisable.

Literature

The code for this substrate in the literature list is *1* (see p. 126).

2. b-ile-glu(pip)-glu-arg-pNA · HCl

substrate for: factor X_a
commercial name: S 2337

Chemical name: N-Benzoyl-L-isoleucyl-L-glutamyl-(γ-piperidyl)-glycyl-
L-ariginine-p-nitroanilide hydrochloride

Formula: ⬡ -CO-Ile-Glu(N)-Glu-Arg-NH-⬡ -NO$_2$ · HCl

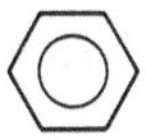

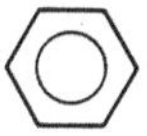

Mol. weight: 801.5

E_{max}: 1.27×10^4 mol^{-1}. l. cm^{-1} (λ_{max}: 316 nm in H$_2$O)

Solubility: 2 mmol. l^{-1} in H$_2$O

Stability: comparable to S 2222

Stock solution
Like for S 2222 but at a three fold higher dilution because of the poor
solubility. Calculations should be made on basis of an E_{max} of 1.27×10^4
instead of 1.28×10^4 mol^{-1}. l. cm^{-1} at 316 nm.

Kinetic data
With activated human factor X this substrate shows a K_m of about 80 μM
(pH 8.0, 37°C. Tris buffer. I 0.20), k_{cat} is 140 sec^{-1} under these conditions. The data for bovine thrombin are comparable. 5 μl/ml of
activated plasma (~ 0.1 pM of factor X_a) is reported to give an adsorbancy change of 0.05 O.D.U./min at a substrate concentration of 0.3 mM.

Literature

The code for this substrate in the literature list is *2* (see p. 126).

3. pglu-gly-arg-pNA · HCl

substrate for: urokinase
commercial name: S 2444.

Chemical name:	L-pyroglutamyl-glycyl-L-arginine-p-nitroanilide hydrochloride.

Formula: pyroglu-gly-arg-NH-⟨◯⟩-NO$_2$ · HCl

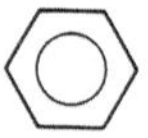

Mol. weight:	498.9
E_{max}:	1.28×10^4 mol^{-1}. l. cm^{-1} (λ_{max}: 316 nm in H$_2$O)
Solubility:	> 10 mmol. l^{-1} in H$_2$O
	3 mmol. l^{-1} in Tris buffer (pH 8.8 I 0.05)
Stability:	comparable to S 2222

Kinetic data

K_m for urokinase is about 50 μM, k_{cat} about 15 sec^{-1}. The concentration of NaCl has a marked influence on the kinetic data. In the range of 0.3–0.7 M the kinetic constants are largely independent of changes in NaCl concentration. Most data are given at 0.05 M of NaCl. This may account for part of the reported variability (G. Wijngaards, personal communication). Trypsin also readily splits this substrate.

Literature

The code for this substrate in the literature list is *3* (see p. 126).

4. b-val-gly-arg-pNA · HCl

substrate for: Urokinase
commercial name: Chromozym UK

Chemical name: N-Benzoyl-L-valyl-glycyl-L-arginine-p-nitroanilide
hydrochloride

Formula: ⟨◯⟩ CO-Val-Gly-Arg-NH-⟨◯⟩-NO₂ · HCl

Mol. weight: 559.1

E_{max}: 1.28×10^{-4} mol^{-1}. l. cm^{-1} (λ_{max}: 323 nm in H_2O)

Solubility: comparable to S 2222

Stability: comparable to S 2222

Remark
The same peptide sequence with a carbobenzoxy N-terminal group is known as Chromozym Try.

Kinetic data
Many of the kinetic data for this substrate are obtained with a first batch that later appeared to be substituted in the arg residue.

K_m : 25 μM.
V_{max} : 8×10^{-7} Mole. min^{-1}. (I.U.)$^{-1}$.

Literature

The code for this substrate in the literature list is *4* (see p. 126).

5. H.D.-val-leu-arg-pNA · 2 HCl

substrate for: Glandular kallikrein
commercial name: S 2226

Chemical name: H-D-valyl-L-leucyl-L-arginine-p-nitroanilide
dihydrochloride

Formula: H-D-val-leu-arg-NH- ⟨◯⟩ -NH$_2$ · 2 HCl

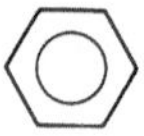

Mol. weight: 579.6

E_{max}: 1.28×10^{-4} mol^{-1}.l.cm^{-1} (λ_{max}: 316 nm in H$_2$O)

Solubility: $\sim$ 40 mmol.l^{-1} in H$_2$O
5 mM in Tris buffer (pH 9.0, I 0.05)

Stability: see S 2222

Kinetic data
Diverse glandular kallikreins at pH around 9 show a K_m for this substrate of $2-4 \times 10^{-5}$ Mol. l^{-1}. V_{max} is given as about 8×10^{-9} mol. min^{-1}. (K.U.)$^{-1}$. For human salivary kallikrein, K_m is reported to be 5×10^{-4} mol. l^{-1}. The substrate is relatively insensitive towards urokinase.

Literature

The code for this substrate in the literature list is 5 (see p. 126).

6. b-pro-phe-arg-pNA · HCl

Substrate for: Plasma Kallikrein
Commercial name: Chromozym PK
                 Chromokallikrein

Chemical name: N-benzoyl-L-propyl-L-phenylalanyl-L-arginine-
                  p-nitroanilide-hydrochloride

Formula: ⬡-CO-Pro-Phe-Arg-NH⬡-NO$_2$ · HCl

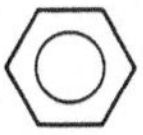

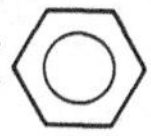

Mol. weight: 679.3

E_{max}: 1.28×10^4 mol^{-1}. l. cm^{-1} (λ_{max}: 316 nm in H$_2$O)

Solubility: 7 mmol. l^{-1} in H$_2$O

Stability: see S 2222

Kinetic data

Plasma kallikrein shows a K_m for this substrate of 10−40 mM at pH around 8.

V_{max} is 1.7×10^{-3} M. min^{-1} per the amount of kallikrein in 1 ml plasma ($\sim$ 2.nmol)

k_{cat} is roughly estimated to be 25 sec.$^{-1}$

Different coagulation factors (II, X_a, XII$_a$) show a K_m of the same or up till 5× higher magnitude. k_{cat} is about 10× smaller. The kinetic parameters for trypsin, urokinase and plasmin are of the same order or magnitude as those for kallikrein.

Literature

The code for this substrate in the literature list is *6* (see p. 126).

7. H-D-pro-phe-arg-pNA · 2 HCl

Substrate for: plasma kallikrein
commercial name: S 2302

Chemical name:	H.D.-Propyl-L-phenylalanine-L-arginine-p-nitroanilide dihydrochloride

Formula: H-D-pro-phe-arg-NH-⟨◯⟩-NO$_2$ · 2 HCl

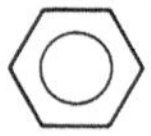

Mol. weight: 611.6

E_{max}: 1.28×10^4 mol^{-1}. l. cm^{-1} (λ_{max}: 316 nm in H$_2$O)

Solubility: $\sim$ 10 mmol. l^{-1} in H$_2$O
5 mmol. l^{-1} in Tris buffer pH 7.8. I 0.05

Stability: see S 2222

Kinetic data

Plasma kallikrein shows a K_m for this substrate of $\sim 2 \times 10^{-4}$ mol. l^{-1} at pH 7.8.

V_{max} is $\sim 6 \times 10^{-6}$ mol. min^{-1} per the amount of kallikrein in 1 ml of plasma (2 nmol).

k_{cat} is roughly estimated to be 10 sec^{-1}.

The kinetic parameters of II$_a$ (bovine), X$_a$, XII$_a$, plasmin, trypsin are of the same order of magnitude. The substrate is relatively unsensitive towards urokinase.

Literature

The code for this substrate in the literature list is 7 (see p. 126).

8. H.D.-phe-pip-arg-pNA · 2 HCl

substrate for: thrombin
commercial name: S 2238

Chemical name: H.D.phenylanlanyl-L-pipecolyl-L-arginine-p-
nitroanilide dihydrochloride

Formula: H.D.-Phe-Pip-Arg-NH-⟨O⟩-NO_2 · 2 HCl

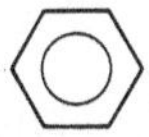

Mol. weight: 625.6

E_{max}: $1.28 \times 10^4 . mol^{-1} . l. cm^{-1}$ (λ_{max}: 316 nm in H_2O)

Solubility: ~ 10 mmol. l^{-1} in H_2O
5 mmol. l^{-1} in Tris buffer (pH 8.3, I 0.15)

Stability: see S 2222

Kinetic data

K_m for thrombin 10 μM (pH 8.3, I 0.15 Tris buffer)
k_{cat}: 100–200 sec^{-1} $k_{cat}/K_m = 5 \times 10^7 . sec^{-1} . M^{-1} .l$
The maximal velocity is $\sim 2 \times 10^{-7}$ mol. min^{-1}. (N.I.H.)U.$^{-1}$
In the presence of large amounts of factor X_a, Soybean Trypsin inhibitor should be used to prevent side reactions.
K_m for plasmin and urokinase is about 1–3 mM, k_{cat} 5–50 sec^{-1}.
Extensive data on kinetic parameters as a function of pH, buffer composition etc. are to be found in (22).
It has been reported that this substrate inhibits the action of factor X_a on prothrombin and chromozym TH by a partial non competitive mechanism.
($K_i \sim 80 \mu$M) (21). From the K_m for factor X_a (35 μM) and k_{cat} ($< 1.sec^{-1}$) it can be seen that this substrate will bind to factor X_a, be it hardly split.

Literature

The code for this substrate in the literature list is *8* (see p. 126).

9. t-gly-pro-arg-pNA · HCl

substrate for: thrombin
commercial name: Chromozym TH
                       Chromothrombin

Chemical name:	N-tosyl-glycyl-L-prolyl-L-arginine-p-nitroanilide hydrochloride

Formula: H_3C-⟨O⟩-Gly-Pro-Arg-NH-⟨O⟩-NO_2 · HCl

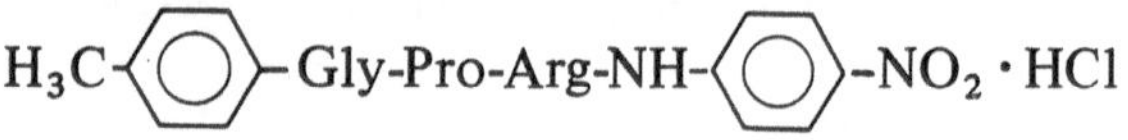

Mol. weight: 639.1

E_{max}: 1.28×10^4 $mol^{-1}.l. cm^{-1}$ (λ_{max}: 323 nm in H_2O)

Solubility: 6 mmol.l^{-1} in Tris buffer

Stability: see S 2222

Kinetic data

Thrombin (human or bovine) splits this substrate in a reaction with a K_m of 400. μmol. l^{-1}

k_{cat}: 100–200 sec^{-1} k_{cat}/K_m 3×10^4 . sec^{-1} . mol^{-1} . l.

Soybean trypsin inhibitor can be used to inhibit factor X_a.

K_m for X_a is 10–50 × higher than for thrombin, k_{cat} is of the same order of magnitude. The same holds for plasmin. Trypsin shows a K_m of ~ 20 μM and a k_{cat} of 75.sec^{-1}.

Extensive and precise data on K_m with thrombin as a function of pH and buffer composition are to be found in (22).

Literature

The code for this substrate in the literature list is *9* (see p. 126).

10. D-ile-pro-arg-pNA · HCl

Substrate: many serine proteases primarily thrombin
Commercial name: S 2288

Chemical name: H-D-isoleucyl-L-propyl-L-arginine-p-nitroanilide-
dihydrochloride

Formula: H-D-ile-pro-arg-NH –⟨◯⟩–NO_2 · 2 HCl

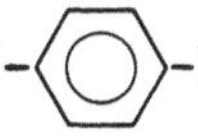

Mol. weight: 577.6

E_{max}: 1.28×10^4 mol^{-1}. l. cm^{-1} (λ_{max}: 316 nm in H_2O)

Solubility: ~ 40 mN in H_2O
~ 10 mM in Tris buffer pH 8.4 I 0.15

Stability: see S 2222

Kinetic data

ENZYME	K_m(M)	k_{cat} (sec^{-1})	k_{cat}/K_m
Thrombin(hum)	3×10^{-6}	120	4×10^7
Thrombin(bov.)	1×10^{-6}	75	7.5×10^7
Factor X_a	2×10^{-3}	110	5.5×10^4
Factor XII_a	4×10^{-4}	23	6×10^4
Plasma kallikrein	1×10^{-3}		
Plasmin	9×10^{-3}	181	2×10^4
Urokinase	2×10^{-4}	16	8×10^4
TPA-1ch	1×10^{-3}	26	2.5×10^4
TPA-2ch	3×10^{-4}	28	9×10^4
C 1s	3×10^{-3}	4	1×10^3
C 2s	6×10^{-4}	2	3×10^3
(37°C. Tris buffer pH 8.4. I 0.15)			

S 2238 is a fairly good substrate for thrombin if a sensitive spectrophotometer is available. At a substrate concentration of $10 \mu M$ thrombin
will act at 77% of its maximal activity. Factor X_a at $\frac{1}{2}$%, Plasmin at
0, 1%, Kallikrein at 1%.

Literature

The code for this substrate in the literature list is *10* (see p. 126).

11. b-phe-leu-arg-pNA

Substrate for: thrombin and other serine proteases
Commercial name: S 2160

Chemical name: N-benzoyl-L-nitrophenylalanyl-L-leucyl-L-arginine-p-
nitroanilide

Formula: ⟨◯⟩–CO-(NO_2)Phe-Val-Arg-NH–⟨◯⟩–$NO_2 \cdot$ HCl

Mol. weight: 681.2

E_{max}: $1.5 \times 10^4 . \, mol^{-1} . \, 1. \, cm^{-1}$ (λ_{max}: 301 nm in H_2O)

Solubility: 1.5 mmol. 1^{-1} in H_2O
0.13 mmol. 1^{-1} in Tris buffer pH 8.0 I 0.15

Kinetic data
Since this was the first substrate generally available many kinetic data
have been obtained. Still we prefer to give only an indication of the
range in which they are to be found.

ENZYME	K_m(M)	k_{cat} (sec^{-1})	k_{cat}/K_m (sec^{-1}. mol^{-1}. l).
Thrombin	1×10^{-4}	6	6×10^4
Plasmin	9×10^{-4}	8	10^4
Trypsin	5×10^{-5}	60	10^4

As a specific substrate for thrombin S 2160 has been replaced by S 2238.
This substrate inhibits factor X_a by a partial uncompetitive mechanism
(K_i, (app): 12.10 mM) (see also no. 8, S 2238 p. 75).

Literature

The code for this substrate in the literature list is *11* (see p. 126).

12. D-val-leu-lys-pNA · 2 HCl

Substrate for: plasmin
Commercial name: S 2251

Chemical name: H-D-valyl-L-leucyl-L-lysine-p-nitroanilide
dihydrochloride

Formula: H-D-val-leu-lys-NH –⟨◯⟩–NO_2 · 2 HCl

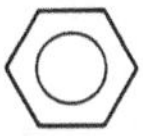

Mol. weight: 551.5

E_{max}: 1.28×10^4 . mol^{-1} . l. cm^{-1} (λ_{max} : 316 nm in H_2O)

Solubility: ~ 40 mmol. l^{-1} in H_2O
~ 10 mmol. l^{-1} in Tris buffer (pH 7.4. I 0.15)

Stability: see S 2222

Kinetic data
Human plasmin: K_m 0.2 mM
k_{cat} 12 sec^{-1}
k_{cat}/K_m 6×10^4 sec^{-1} . M^{-1} l.
(pH 7.4 Tris buffer I 0.15 37°C)

The substrate is insensitive to kallikrein (glandular and plasma-) and urokinase as well as to thrombin (human and bovine) and factor X_a, Glu-Plasminogen SK, Val 442-Plasmogen-SK, Lys-Plasmin SK, Val 442-Plasmin SK and Plasmin B chain SK show K_m's varying from 2–8 × 10^{-4} M, k_{cat} of 30–50 sec^{-1}, k_{cat}/K_m of ~ 10^5 sec^{-1} . M^{-1} . l. Plasmogen SK shows a K_m of 2×10^{-4} M, $k_{cat} = 1$ sec^{-1} (23). Trypsin readily splits this substrate.

Literature

The code for this substrate in the literature list is *12* (see p. 126).

13. t-gly-pro-lys-pNA · HCl

substrate for: plasmin
Commercial name: chromozym PL
                 chromoplasmin

Chemical name: N-tosyl-glycyl-L-propyl-L-arginine-p-nitroanilide
                 hydrochloride

Formula: $H_3C-\langle\bigcirc\rangle-gly\text{-}pro\text{-}lys\text{-}NH-\langle\bigcirc\rangle-NO_2 \cdot HCl$

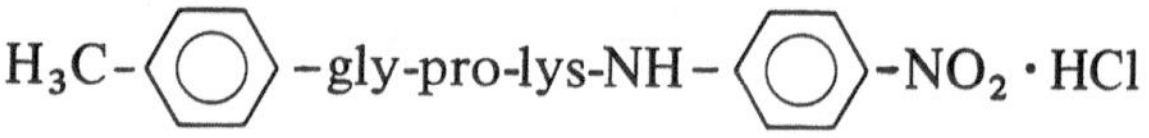

Mol. weight: 611.1

E_{max} : 1.28×10^4 mol.$^{-1}$. cm^{-1} (λ_{max} : 323 nm in H_2O)

Solubility: 7 mmol. l^{-1} in Tris buffer

Stability: see S 2222

Kinetic data

	K_m (M)	k_{cat} (sec^{-1})	k_{cat}/K_m (sec^{-1} mol^{-1} . l)
Plasmin	2.5×10^{-4}	50	2×10^3
Glu-Plasminogen-SK	5×10^{-4}	30	6×10^4
Urokinase	2×10^{-3}	40	2×10^4
Thrombin (bov)	2×10^{-5}	20	1×10^6
Thrombin (hum)	5×10^{-5}	30	6×10^5
Factor X$_a$ (bov)	—	—	1×10^5
Trypsin	1.5×10^{-5}	15	1×10^6

It is clear that this substrate is readily split by coagulation factors.

Literature

The code for this substrate in the literature list is *13* (see p. 126).

14. cmprop-arg-pro-tyr-pNA · HCl

Substrate for: chymotrypsin
Commercial name: S 2586

Chemical name: 3-Carbomethoxyproprionyl-L-arginyl-L-propyl-L-
                       tyrosine-p-nitroanilide hydrochloride

Formula: $CH_3-O-CH_2-CH_2-CO$-arg-pro-tyr-NH-⟨◯⟩- 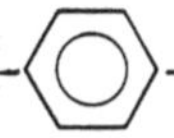
                NO_2 · HCl

Mol. weight: 705.3

E_{max}: $1.28 \times 10^4 . mol^{-1}. l. cm^{-1} (\lambda_{max}: 316\,nm$ in $H_2O)$

Solubility: 10 mmol. l^{-1} in H_2O
            2 mmol. l^{-1} in 0.03 M Tris buffer (pH 8.3, I 0.4)

Stability: see S 2222

Kinetic data

$K_m \sim 5 \times 10^{-5}$ M
$k_{cat} \sim 140\,sec^{-1}$
$k_{cat}/K_m \sim 3 \times 10^5\,sec^{-1}, mol^{-1}. l$ (Tris. pH 8.3. I 0.4)
The substrate is insensitive to factor X_a, kallikreins (glandular or plasma-), plasmin, thrombin, trypsin, urokinase and hardly is split by granulocyte elastase and cathepsin G.

Literature

The code for this substrate in the literature list is *14* (see p. 126).

15. pglu-pro-val-pNA

substrate for: granulocyte elastase
commercial name: S 2484

Chemical name:	L-pyroglutamyl-L-propyl-L-valine--p-nitroanilide hydrochloride

Formula: p.glu-pro-val-NH$-\langle\bigcirc\rangle-NO_2$

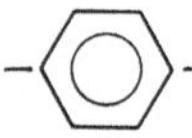

Mol. weight: 445.5

E_{max}: $1.28 \times 10^4 . \text{mol}^{-1}. 1. \text{cm}^{-1} (\lambda_{max}:$ 316 nm in $H_2O)$

Solubility: 1 mmol. 1^{-1} in H_2O, 8 mmol in H_2O + 25% DMSO
0.3 mmol. 1^{-1} in 0.03 M Tris buffer (pH 8.3, I 0.3)
2 mmol. 1^{-1} in the same buffer with 8% DMSO

Stability: see S 2222

Kinetic data
K_m of granulocyte elastase for this enzyme is 3×10^{-4} mol. 1^{-1}, $k_{cat} \sim$ 9 sec^{-1}, k_{cat}/K_m $3 \times 10^4 . \text{sec}^{-1}. \text{mol}^{-1}. 1$
(determined in the above mentioned buffer with 8% DMSO).
The substrate is insensitive to factor X_a, kallikrein (glandular − or plasma −), plasmin, thrombin, trypsin, urokinase; pancreas elastase and chymotrypsin split this enzyme slowly ($<$ 1% of the granulocyte elastase).

Literature

The code for this substrate in the literature list is *15* (see p. 126).

III.5. Fluorogenic substrates

Instead of the chromogenic *p*-Nitroaniline group various other groups can be attached to an oligopeptide. If these groups have specific fluorescence characteristics their liberation by amidolytic enzymes can be followed in a fluorimeter. Fluorimetry is known to be about ten fold more sensitive than spectrophotometry and this may be a useful property in designing sensitive tests (see p. 44). Still the use of fluorogenic substrates has not at this moment found widespread use.

Fluorogenic leaving groups

Five different fluorogenic groups have been used to monitor oligopeptide splitting. The longest known are the naphtylamines (Table III.5, no. 1 and 2) (24, 25) that, because of their established carcinogenicity probably will not find widespread use.

The groups most extensively studied are the coumarin derivatives (Table III.5 no. 3 and 4) to which a separate paragraph will be dedicated. The 7-amino-4-methylcoumarin (MCA) compound has been studied systematically by the group of Iwanaga and used as the basis of a number of fluorimetric assays (refs. 26–31) further details of which are to be found in Chapter IV. Because of its importance a detailed description of the use of this type of substrates follows separately.

Other groups used as fluorophore in oligopeptides are aminoisophtalic acid (32) and 5-amino isopthalic acid dimethylester (33).

III.6. General principles of fluorogenic peptide substrates with 7-amino-4-methyl-coumarine as a leaving group (Contributed by S. Iwanaga, H. Kato, T. Morita, T. Sugo, Y. Ohno, M. Ohki, K. Takada and S. Sakakibara.)

Peptide amides of 7-amino-4-methylcoumarin (MCA), originally developed for the sensitive assay for α-chymotrypsin (34) and an aminopeptidase (35), have also proven useful for the assay of proteases including elastase (36), X-propyl dipeptidase (37) and pyroglutamyl peptidase (38). This assay method is more sensitive than the chromogenic assay, because the reaction product, 7-amino-4-methylcoumarin is highly fluorescent.

To extend further the availability of fluorogenic substrates, we have newly synthesized 41 peptidyl-MCA's and tested them for their possible use as specific substrates for assay of proteolytic enzymes with limited specificity (26). The results indicate that the peptidyl-MC substrate, which fits preferentially the specificity requirements of α-thrombin,

Table III.5.   Fluorogenic leaving groups.

1.		2-naphtylamine (βNA)
2.		4-methoxy-2-naphylamine (MβNA) (32)
3.		7-amino-4-methylcoumarin (MCA) (34, 26)
4.		7-amino-4-trifluorocarbon coumarine (TFCA)
5.		5-amino-isophtalic acid dimethylester (AIE) (33)

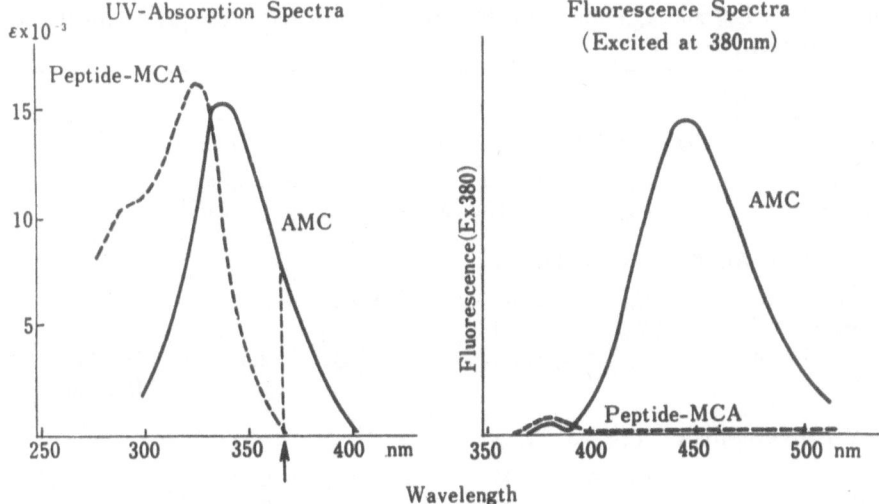

Fig. III.1. Ultraviolet and fluorescence spectra of peptide MCA and AMC.

Factor X_a, kallikreins, plasmin, horseshoe crab clotting enzyme and urokinase, is valuable for specific enzyme assay. This paragraph describes a general principle, method and application of the fluorogenic substrate assay methods for proteinases in blood coagulation, kallikrein-kinin and fibrinolysis systems.

A protease with limited specificity hydrolyzes a peptide-MCS substrate, releasing 7-amino-4-methylcoumarin (AMC) as follows

$$X-Y-Z-Arg-NH- \text{(MCA)} + H_2O \xrightarrow{\ enzyme\ }$$

MCA ... CH₃

$$X-Y-Z-Arg-OH + H_2N- \text{(AMC)}$$

AMC CH₃

Because the reaction product, AMC, is highly fluorescent, the rate at which AMC is released can be measured fluorometrically with excitation at 380 nm and emission at 440 nm (Fig. III.1). The amount of AMC released can also be estimated photometrically at 370 nm (Fig. III.1). Release of AMC can be followed on a recorder (initial-rate method) or read by terminating the enzyme reaction with acetic acid (end-point method).

Table III.6. K_m and k_{cat} values for the interaction of serine esterases with fluorogenic substrates.

MβNA (4-methyl-)2-naphtylamine

---

1. Gly-Arg-βNA (Bachem, Liestal, Switzerland) (24, 25, 39)

| Plasmin | $K_m = 1.7 \times 10^{-3}$ M | $k_{cat} = 0.03 \sec^{-1}$ |
| Urokinase | $K_m = 7.5 \times 10^{-3}$ M | $k_{cat} = 3.6 \sec^{-1}$ |

2. Boc-Val-Gly-Arg-βNA (24, 25, 39)

Plasmin	$K_m = 1.6$ mM	$k_{cat} = 0.11 \sec^{-1}$
Urokinase	$K_m = 1.1$ mM	$k_{cat} = 0.5 \sec^{-1}$
Tissue activator	$K_m = 0.5$ mM	$V_{max} = 2.4 \times 10^{-12}$ M/CTA Un/min

3. H-Val-Gly-Arg-βNA (24, 25, 39)

| Plasmin | $K_m = 0.9$ mM | $k_{cat} = 0.05 \sec^{-1}$ |
| Urokinase | $K_m = 0.6$ mM | $k_{cat} = 0.8 \sec^{-1}$ |

4. Cbz-Gly-Pro-Arg-βNA (40)

| Thrombin | $K_m = 83 \,\mu$M |

5. Cbz-Ala-Ala-Lys-MβNA (41)

| Plasmin | $K_m = 870 \,\mu$M |

AIE 5 amino isophtalic acid dimethyl ester

---

6. H-D-Phe-Pro-Arg-AIA (Dade) (32)
   (anal. S 2338)

| Thrombin | $K_m = 54 \,\mu$M |

7. H-D-Val-Leu-Lys-AIA (Dade) (42, 43)
   (anal. S 2251)

| Plasmin | $K_m = 250 \,\mu$M |

TFCA 7 amino-4-trifluorocarbonylcoumarin

---

8. Cbz-Gly-Gly-Arg-TFCA (44)

| Trypsin | $K_m = 180 \,\mu$M | $k_{cat} = 135 \sec^{-1}$ |
| Urokinase | $K_m = 190 \,\mu$M | $V_{max} = 3 \times 10^{-5} =$ M/min/IU |

9. H-D-Ala-Leu-Lys-TFCA (45, 46)

| Plasmin | $K_m = 620 \,\mu$M | $V_{max} = 0.067 \,\mu$M/min/CTA U |

   H-D-Val-Leu-Lys-TFCA

| Plasmin | $K_m = 560 \,\mu$M | $V_{max} = 0.088 \,\mu$M/min/CTA U |

(44)

Table III.6. continued

MCA   7-Amino-4-methylcoumarine

---

10. Glu-Gly-Arg-MCA   (28)

Urokinase $K_m = 320\,\mu M$ $k_{cat} > 10\,sec^{-1}$

11. Boc-Ile-Glu-Gly-Arg-MCA   (26, 28)

Factor X_a $K_m = 160\,\mu M$ $k_{cat} \geqslant 4\,sec^{-1}$

12. Cbz-Gly-Gly-Arg-MCA   (47, 44)

Trypsin $K_m = 330\,\mu M$ $60\,sec^{-1}$
Thrombin $K_m = 100\,\mu M$ $\geqslant 300\,sec^{-1}$
Plasmin $K_m = 450\,\mu M$ $10\,M/min/CTA\ U$
Urokinase $K_m = 150\,\mu M$ $\geqslant 900\,sec^{-1}$

13. Boc-Leu-Gly-Arg-MCA   (48, 26)

Limulus enzyme $K_m = 27\,\mu M$ $V_{max} = 4.8\,\mu M/min\ mg$

14. Boc-Ser-Gly-Arg-MCA   (48)

Limulus enzyme $K_m = 24\,\mu M$ $V_{max} = 4.3\,\mu M/min\ mg$

15. Pro-Phe-Arg-MCA   (28)

Plasma
  kallikrein (bov) $K_m = 600\,\mu M$ $V_{max} = 3\,\mu M/min\ A\,280 = 1.0$
Urinary kallikrein $K_m = 200\,\mu M$ $V_{max} = 30\,\mu M/min\ mg$
Hageman factor $K_m = 50\,\mu M$ $k_{cat} = 2\,sec^{-1}$
Pancreatic
  kallikrein K_m $V_{max} = 12\,\mu M/min\ A\,280 = 1.0$

16. Cbz-Pro-Phe-Arg-MCA

Plasma kallikrein $K_m = 500\,\mu M$ $V_{max} = 7.2\,\mu M/min\ A\,280 = 1.0$
Urinary kallikrein $K_m = 170\,\mu M$ $V_{max} = 7.5\,\mu M/min\ mg$
Pancreatic
  kallikrein $K_m = 180\,\mu M$ $V_{max} = 4.6\,\mu M/min\ A\,280 = 1.0$

17. Cbz-Phe-Arg-MCA

Plasma
  kallikrein (bov) $K_m = 250\,\mu M$ $V_{max} = 8.0\,\mu M/min\ A\,280 = 1.0$
Urinary
  kallikrein (hum) $K_m = 300\,\mu M$ $V_{max} = 1.1\,\mu M/min\ mg$
Pancreatic
  kallikrein (hog) $K_m = 500\,\mu M$ $V_{max} = 0.3\,\mu M/min\ A\,280 = 1.0$

18. Boc-Val-Pro-Arg-MCA   (28)

Thrombin (bov) $K_m = 20\,\mu M$ $k_{cat} \geqslant 30\,sec^{-1}$

Table III.6. continued

---

19. Boc-Phe-Ser-Arg-MCA (28)

Factor XII_a

20. Boc-Leu-Thr-Arg-MCA

Factor XII_a

21. Boc-Val-Leu-Lys-MCA (46)

Plasmin (bov)	K_m	= 250 μM	V_{max}	= 1.5 μM/min mg
Plasmin (hum)	K_m	= 800 μM	V_{max}	= 3.7 μM/min mg

22. Boc-Glu-Lys-Lys-MCA

Plasmin (bov)	K_m	= 700 μM	V_{max}	= 1.9 μM/min mg
Plasmin (hum)	K_m	= 800 μM	V_{max}	= 3.7 μM/min mg

23. Boc-Gly-Lys-Lys-MCA (28)

24. Boc-Phe-Glu-Lys-Lys-MCA

Plasmin (bov)	K_m	= 400 μM	V_{max}	= 0.23 μM/min mg

25. Succinoyl-Ala-Phe-Lys-MCA (47)

Plasmin	K_m	= 400 μM	V_{max}	= 370 μM/min CTA unit
Urokinase	K_m	= 800 μM	V_{max}	= 62 μM/min mg

26. MeOSuc-Ala-Phe-Lys-MCA

Plasmin	K_m	= 440 μM	V_{max}	= 470 μM/min CTA unit

27. Boc-Leu-Ser-Thr-Arg-MCA (49)

Protein C (bov)	K_m	= 330 μM	k_{cat}	= 8.4 sec^{-1}

III.7. Thioesters

Apart from paranitro anilide other groups can be attached to polypeptides that can be split of by serine proteases and then monitored spectrophotometrically.

Thioesters of specific amino acids and polypeptides are split by chymotrypsin, elastase and trypsin (50, 51, 52). The thiol that arises upon splitting can be determined continuously if 4,4'-dithiodipyridine (Aldrithiol-4) is present, as these two substances react to form 4-dithiodipyridine which has the extremely high extinction coefficient of 19 800 mol^{-1} . l. cm^{-1} at 324 nm.

McRae *et al.* (53) recently reported studies in which a large series of thiolesters were tested for their suitability as substrates of factors II_a, X_a, IX_a, XI_a, XII_a and a plasma kallikrein of bovine origin.

Apart from variations in the amino acid part of the substrate the thiol residues can also be varied. Isobutylthiol and Benzylthiol have been used.

Also it is possible to substitute the oxygen in an amide link between two amino acids by a sulfer. This opens the interesting possibility to mimic amino acid sequences at both sides of a vulnerable site. It appears that not only the N terminal part – the part that varies in paranitroanilide containing substrates – but also the leaving group determines the kinetic constants (and thus the selectivity) of a given substrate.

Amino acid and dipeptide thioester substrates show a k_{cat}/K_m in the range of $10^4 - 10^5$ for factor X_a and the same or lower for factor XII_a. About half of the substrates show a k_{cat}/K_m of between 10^5 and 10^6 for factors XI_a and prekallikrein. For thrombin and trypsin the efficiency constant may be in the $10^5 - 10^6$ range. No simple high selectivities for one coagulation factor are found however. Tripeptides are split with an efficiency constant of $10^5 - 10^6$ by thrombin, $> 10^6$ by trypsin, $10^4 - 10^5$ by factors X_a and XI_a. Among these there are some that are split by factor IX_a, but with kinetic constants in the same range as factors X_a or XI_a, so that the specificity is low.

A typical reaction mixture consists of:

20 ml   0.10 M Hepes buffer pH 7,5 containing 0.01 MCaCl$_2$ and 9.8% v/v DMSO, containing substrate to the required concentration.

0.150 ml   of a 2 mM solution of 4,4^1-dithiodipyridine

0.050 ml   of enzyme solution.

The reaction rate is monitored at 324 nM.

The precise substrate concentration is checked by adding 20 μl of a 10^{-5} M trypsin solution at the end of the experiment. Trypsin is universally active against these substrates, so this makes the reaction run to completion.

III.8. Substrates for electrochemical determinations

A list of substrates that can be used in electrochemical determinations is given in Table III.7. It is reported that the p-amino-diphenylamine (pADA) group on tripeptides yields substrates with kinetic constant that differ only insignificantly from the same peptides with p-Nitroanilide

Table III.7. Substrates for electrochemical determinations.

D.L. Benzoylarginine HCl	Trypsin	DL. BAPADA
H.D. Phe-pip-Arg-pADA · 2 HCl	Thrombin	S-2497
H.D. Val-Leu-Lys-pADA · 2 HCl	Plasmin	S-2644
Bz-Ile-Glu(pip)-Gly-Arg-pADA · 2 HCl	FX$_a$	S-2646
H.D. Pro-Phe-Arg-pADA	Kallikrein Pl.	S-2648
H.D.-Val-Leu-Arg-pADA	Kallikrein U	S-2649

groups. S 2421 (H-D-Phe-pip-arg-4MeO-napthlamine) is an interesting substrate in that its leaving group can be assessed both spectrophotometrically and electrochemically. With the use of this substrate it could be shown that both procedures measure essentially the same process. (54) These substrates are usually added by solving them in dimethylsulfoxide (DMSO) first and then adding the solution to a Tris-HCl-buffer of desired composition. A suitable buffer is Tris/HCl 0.025 M, NaCl 0.12 M, Glycine 0.05 M, DMSO 5% w/w, pH 8.2. (54–57).

III.9. Luminogenic substrates

In luminogenic substrates the enzyme to be determined splits off a luminiscent leaving group from a synthetic peptide substrate. The luminogenic substrates described until now all contain as luminophoric group isoluminolamide (IL) (57, 58).

isoluminolamide (IL):

The principle of the luminogenic assay is the following:

step 1:

step 2:

Table III.8.   Luminogenic substrates.

Substrate	Enzyme	$k_{cat}(\sec^{-1})$	Detection limit(ng)
Boc-Ala-Ala-Phe-IL	chymotrypsin	0.054	230
Z-Ala-Ala-Phe-IL	chymotrypsin	0.43	27
AGlO-Ala-Ala-Ala-Phe-IL	chymotrypsin	0.22	0.1
Z-Phe-Pro-Arg-IL	trypsin	31.7	0.08
AGlO-Ala-Phe-Pro-Arg-IL	trypsin	1.5	0.01
Z-Phe-Pro-Arg-IL	thrombin	4.3	1.3
AGlO-Ala-Phe-Pro-Arg-IL	thrombin	0.05	0.5

The isoluminolamide production is determined by monitoring light emission resulting from the addition of hematin and hydrogen peroxide to alkaline sample mixtures.

To determine IL levels in the presence of the unreacted luminogenic substrate, it is necessary to subtract the total background emission of substrate plus oxidant from the total light emission observed in the reaction mixture containing enzyme, substrate and IL, this is a serious limitation to the sensitivity of the method. To reduce this problem the luminogenic substrates are bound to a solid matrix (Affi-gel:AGlO). After incubation of the enzyme with the substrate suspension the unreacted substrate can be removed by centrifugation and the IL produced determined by the assay of the supernatant.

The incubation of the enzyme with the substrate is usually carried out at 22°C in sodium phosphate (0.05 M, pH 7.8). In the case of a soluble substrate the incubation mixture also contains 10% DMSO. After 5 minutes incubation the immobilized unreacted substrate is removed by centrifugation and 25 μl aliquots of supernatant or incubation mixture (in the case of a soluble substrate) are added to 235 μl NaOH (50 mM, pH 12.6) and 20 μl hematin (6 μM) in Na_2CO_3 (0.1 M, pH 10.5). Light emission is initiated by injecting 20 μl H_2O_2 (90 mM).

References

1. Seegers WH, Landaburu RH: Am J Physiol 191:167−174 (1957)
2. Gaffney PJ, Lord K, Brasher M, Kirkwood TBL: Thromb Res 10:549−556 (1977)
3. Troll W, Sherry S, Wachman J: J Biol Chem 208:85−95 (1954)
4. Gaffney PJ: *In* Chromogenic Peptide Substrates; Chemistry and Clinical Usage. Scully MF, Kakkar VV (eds). Churchill Livingstone, London, 1979, pp 42−49
5. Blow DM, Janin J, Ghothia C: Nature 249:54−55 (1974)
6. Aurell L, Friberger P, Karlsson G: Thromb Res 11:595−609 (1977)
7. Blombäck B, Blombäck M, Olsson PI: Thromb Res 1:267−278 (1972)
8. Svendsen L, Blombäck M, Blombäck B, Olsson PI: Thromb Res 1:267−278 (1972)

9. Suomela H, Blombäck M, Blombäck B: Thromb Res 10:267–281 (1977)
10. Elödi S: Personal communication
11. Østerud B: Personal communication
12. Rosing J, Tans G, Govers-Riemslag JWP, Zwaal RFA, Hemker HC: J Biol Chem 255:274–283 (1980)
13. Geratz JD, Tidwell RR: *In* Chemistry and Biology of Thrombin. Lundblad RL, Fenton JW, Mann KG (eds). Ann Arbor Science Publishers Inc., Ann Arbor, 1977, pp 179–196
14. Kettner C, Shaw E: *In* Chemistry and Biology of Thrombin. Lundblad RL, Fenton JW, Mann KG (eds). Ann Arbor Science Publishers Inc., Ann Arbor, 1977, pp 129–143
15. Geratz JD: Thrombosis et Diathesis Haemorrh 23:486–499 (1970)
16. Markwardt F, Landmann H, Walsmann P: Eur J Biochem 6:502–506 (1968)
17. Stürzebecher J, Markwardt F, Richter P, Voigt B, Wagner G, Walsmann P: Pharmazie 31:458–461 (1976)
18. Okamoto S, Hijikata A, Kinjo K, Kikumoto R, Ohkubu K, Tonomura S, Tamao Y: Kobe J Med Sci 21:43–51 (1975)
19. Jackson C: Thrombosis and Haemostasis 41:458–459 (1979)
20. Enzyme Structure and Mechanism. Fersht A. W.H. Freeman and Co., San Francisco, 1977, pp 96 a.f. pp 274 a.f.
21. Orthner CL, Morris S, Kosov DP: Thromb Res 23:533–539 (1981)
22. Lottenberg R, Christensen U, Jackson CM, Coleman PL: Meth Enzymol 80. Part C Proteolytic enzymes: 341–361 (1981)
23. Wohl RC, Summaria L, Robbins KC: J Biol Chem 255:2005–2013 (1980)
24. Nieuwenhuizen W, Wijngaards G, Groenveld E: Anal Biochemistry 83:143–148 (1977)
25. Nieuwenhuizen W, Wijngaard G, Groenveld E: Thromb Res 11:87–89 (1977)
26. Morita T, Kato H, Iwanaga S, Takada K, Kimura T, Sakakibara S: J Biochem 82:1495–1498 (1978)
27. Harada T, Morita T, Iwanaga S: J Med Enz (in Japanese) 3:43–60 (1978)
28. Iwanaga S, Morita T, Kato H, Harada T, Adachi N, Sugo T, Maruyama I, Takada K, Kimara T, Sakakibara, S: *In* Kinins-II, Biochemistry, Pathophysiology, and Clinical Aspects. Fujii S, Moriya H, Suzuki T (eds). Plenum Publishing Corp., New York, 1978, pp. 147–163
29. Kato H, Sugo T, Ikari N, Hashimoto N, Maruyama I, Han YN, Iwanaga S, Fujii S: *In* Kinins II, Systemic Proteases and Cellular Functions. Fujii S, Moriya H, Suzuki T (eds). Plenum Publishing Corp., New York, 1978, pp. 19–37
30. Harada T, Ohki M, Niwa M, Iwanaga S: Thrombos Haemostas 42:109 (1979)
31. Iwanaga S, Kato H, Maruyama I, Adachi N, Ohno Y, Takada K, Kimura T, Sakakibara S: Thrombos Haemostas 42:49 (1979)
32. Mitchell GA, Garguilo RJ, Huseby RM, Lawson DE, Pochron SP, Sehuanes JA: Thromb Res 13:47–52 (1979)
33. Huseby RM, Mitchell GA, Pochron S, Gargiulo RJ, Hudson PM: *In* New Pathways in Laboratory Medicine. Rosalki S (ed). Hans Huber Publishers, Bern, 1978, pp 50–61
34. Zimmerman, M, Yurewicz EC, Patel G: Anal Biochem 70:258–262 (1976)
35. Kanaoka Y, Takahashi T, Nakayama H: Chem Pharm Bull 25:362–363 (1977)
36 Zimmerman M, Ashe B, Yurewicz EC, Patel G: Anal Biochem 78:47–51 (1977)
37. Kato T, Nagatsu T, Kimura T, Sakakibara S: Seikagaku (in Japanese) 49:990–997 (1977)
38. Fujiwara K, Tsuru D: J Biochem 83:1145–1149 (1978)
39. Nieuwenhuizen W. Wijngaards G, Groenveld E: Heamostasis 7:146–149 (1978)
40. Mitchell GA, Hudson PM, Huseby RF, Pochron SP, Gargiulo RJ: Thromb Res 12:219–225 (1978)

41. Clavin SA, Bobbitt JL, Shuman RT, Smithwick EL Jr: Anal Biochem 80:355–365 (1977)
42. Pochron SP, Mitchell GA, Albareda I, Huseby RM, Gargiulo RJ: Thromb Res 13:733–739 (1978)
43. Lawson DE, Mitchell GA, Huseby RM: Thromb Res 14:323–332 (1979)
44. Smith RE, Bissell ER, Mitchell AR, Pearson KW: Thromb Res 17:393–402 (1980)
45. Friberger P, Claeson G, Knös M, Aurell L, Arielly S, Simonsson R: In: Progress in Chemical Fibrinolysis and Thrombolysis, Vol. 4, Davidson JF (ed). Churchill Livingstone, Edinburgh, 1979, pp 149–153
46. Kato H, Adachi N, Ohno Y, Iwanaga S, Takada K, Sakakibara S: J Biochem 88:183–190 (1980)
47. Pierzchala PA, Dorn CP, Zimmerman M: Biochem J 183:555–559 (1979)
48. Iwanaga S, Morita T, Harada T, Nakamura S, Niwa M, Takada K, Kimura T, Sakakibara S: Haemostasis 7:183–188 (1978)
49. Ohno Y, Kato H, Morita T, Iwanaga S, Takada K, Sakakibara S, Stenflo J: J Biochem 90:1387–1395 (1981)
50. Farmer DA, Hageman JH: J Biol Chem 250:7366–7372 (1975)
51. Castillo MJ, Nakajima K, Zimmerman M, Powers JC: Anal Biochem 99:53–64 (1979)
52. Green GDJ, Shaw E: Anal Biochem 93:223–226 (1979)
53. McRae B, Nakajima B, Travis J, Powers JC: Biochemistry 19:3973–3978 (1980)
54. Daraio de Peuriot M, Nigretto JM, Jozefowicz M: Thromb Res 22:303–308 (1981)
55. Daraio de Peuriot M, Nigretto JM, Jozefowicz M: Thromb Res 17:611–622 (1980)
56. Daraio de Peuriot M, Nigretto JM, Jozefowicz M: Thromb Res 19:647–654 (1980)
57. Daraio de Peuriot M, Nigretto JM, Jozefowicz M: Thromb Res 20:299–306 (1980)
58. Branchini BR, Hermes JD, Salituro FG, Post NJ, Claeson G: Anal Bioch 111:87–89 (1981)
59. Branchini BR, Salituro FG, Hermes JD, Post NJ: Biochem Biophys Res Comm 97:334–339 (1980)

IV. Determinations that can be carried out with chromogenic substrates

Summary

This chapter gives a review of the determinations of clotting- and fibrin-olytic factors and their inhibitors known until medio 1982. It is not complete in the sense that every known variant of every determination has been listed. It has been our aim to select for each different factor (or cofactor or inhibitor) a determination that either in our hands or as reported in the literature shows satisfactory results. This does not mean that the method is optimal. In fact on basis of theory and experience objections can often be readily formulated. In our opinion it is better, at this stage, to give a review of the practical possibilities available than to stress possible shortcomings of the existing methods.

When available we tried to include information necessary to allow carrying out the experiments.

IV.1. Thrombin and derived determinations

Thrombin can be measured with the following substrates:

a. H-D-Phe-Pip-Arg-pNA · HCl (S2238)
b. N-tos-Gly-Pro-Arg-pNA · HCl (chromozym TH)
c. N-benz-NO$_2$Phe-Val-Arg-pNA · HCl (S2160)

These substrates are split not only by α-thrombin but also by β-thrombin, γ-thrombin, meizothrombin and coagulase-thrombin. The specific activities of the various forms of thrombin towards different chromogenic substrates may vary (1, 2). Much less variation is encountered however with artificial substrates than with the natural substrates such as fibrino-gen or factors V, VIII, XIII and platelets. Therefore there need not be a fixed relation between biological and amidolytic activity in different thrombin preparations.

Thrombin estimation is at the basis of a number of prothrombin, antithrombin III (c.q. heparin cofactor) and heparin (c.q. antiheparins, like platelet factor 4) determinations. Also the factors constituting the prothrombinase complex can be measured by assessing the velocity of activation of prothrombin. This leads to factor V and platelet factor 3 determinations.

1.1. Thrombin

Thrombin activity can be assessed in the following medium:

Tris/HCl pH 7.8	20 mM
NaCl	100 mM
Ovalbumin	0,5 mg/ml
Soybean Trypsin inhibitor	5 μg/ml
S 2238 ·	272 μM

Soybean trypsin inhibitor needs only be added if factor X_a can be expected to be present in such a quantity as to cause significant splitting of the substrate. Ovalbumin (or carbowax) addition is especially useful when purified systems are studied because then the low protein-concentration can cause rapid denaturation of the active proteins present a.o. by adsorbtion to cuvette walls etc. The property of thrombin to stick to glass makes it almost impossible to use glass cuvettes repeatedly unless thoroughly cleaned in strong acid. Disposable cuvettes are to be preferred therefore.

The reaction velocity measured is best compared to the velocities obtained with dilutions of an (active site-titrated) thrombin standard. As argued before this will not guarantee standardisation of the biological activities of a particular thrombin preparation.

As a first approximation it can be said that at 37°C, 10^{-10} M of thrombin will cause an optical density change of 5 absorbancy units per minute in the system described above. For the expression of the concentration of thrombin different units are used. The equivalences are listed in Table IV.1.

1.2. Prothrombin

Measuring prothrombin amounts to measuring thrombin after suitable activation. The choice of an activator is crucial here. Non-physiological activators like snake venoms (Taipan snake, Echis carinatus) and staphylocoagulase will usually activate both decarboxy-prothrombin (i.e. the abnormal prothrombin present during oral anticoagulant therapy, also called PIVKA) as well as normal prothrombin. Hence these activators are unsuitable for the estimation of the level of functional prothrombin in vitamin K deficiency (i.e. also in various forms of liver disease) or during oral anticoagulation. The only known activator that differentiates

Table IV.1. Comparison of thrombin concentrations (3)

1 NIH unit	$= 0.324 \pm 0.073\,\mu g$
1 NIH unit	$= (8.85 \pm 2.0)\,10^{-12}\,\text{Mole} = 8.85 \pm 2.01\,\text{p Mole}$
1 μg	$= 27.3 \times 10^{-12}\,\text{Mole} = 27.3\,\text{p Mole}$
1 μg	$= 3.09 \pm 0.57\,\text{NIH units}$
1 p Mole	$= 36.6 \times 10^{-9}\,g = 36.6\,g$
1 p Mole	$= (11.3 \pm 2.8)\,10^{-3}\,\text{NIH units}$
1 IOWA unit	$= 0.83\,\text{NIH unit}$
1 WHO unit	$= 0.56\,\text{NIH unit}$

1 ml of plasma can potentially generate about 1.5×10^{-9} Mole i.e. 1500 pMole or about 17.5 NIH units of thrombin.

between the two species is the physiological prothrombinase consisting of factor X_a, factor V and a suitable phospholipid, which is the activator used by Kirchhof *et al.* (1978) (4). This method is specific for normal prothrombin, and independent of factor V and factor X levels in the plasma. It can be made independent of heparin by the addition of poly-brene. A form of this test is commercialised by Boehringer Mannheim. It can be automated.

In the method by Bergström and Egberg (6) prothrombinase is generated in the sample by the addition of Russell's Viper Venom (RVV) and phospholipid. Consequently the outcome is dependent on the factor X and factor V content in the plasma. There is a high correlation between the outcome of this test in plasmas of orally anticoagulated patients and the conventional thrombotest method as well as with a specific coagulation assay for factor X as would be expected. The test can be automatized (LKB 8600 reaction rate analyses) as can the other tests for prothrombin that are described below. Heparin inhibition can be overcome by the addition of polybrene in the test (5). Bergström and Egberg (6) also describe a prothrombin estimation using Ecarin (Echis carinatus venom). Correlation with conventional clotting assays in control of oral anticoagulation is poor, as would be expected because Ecarin will activate the decarboxy-prothrombin induced by the treatment as well as the normal prothrombin.

Two first generation tests have been published. That of Bergström and Blombäck (7) (1974) uses a partially purified mixture of coagulation factors as a source of prothrombinase. This mixture causes a background activity of 10–20% of that of normal plasma. The tests are heparin inhibited, fibrinogen inhibits as well. Axelsson e.a. (8) (1976) use thromboplastin and endogenous factors V, VII and X as a prothrombin activator. The method consequently is not specific for factor II. It is also hampered by fibrin formation and other turbidities ensuing from the reaction.

A satisfying setup for measuring prothrombin is the following from (4)

sample (undiluted plasma sample)	$1-4\,\mu l$
phospholipid suspension 50 mg/ml in buffer	$10\,\mu l$
factor X_a preparation 50 U/ml in buffer	$10\,\mu l$
CaCl$_2$ 100 mM	$40\,\mu l$
Buffer, 75 mM tris HCl; 75 mM NaCl pH 7.8	$320\,\mu l$
incubation for 120 sec. Then add:	
S 2238 (5 mM)	$20\,\mu l$

$1\,\mu l$ of normal plasma will cause a reaction velocity of about 0.015 absorbancy units per min in this system.

Although standardisation on the velocity of substrate conversion is in principle possible slight variations in temperature, pH etc. may substantially influence the velocity, so standardisation against a standard normal plasma is to be preferred.

It has been observed that thrombin generation by factor X_a (plus phospholipid and factor V) is inhibited markedly by the presence of chromogenic substrates for thrombin (9). This hampers the direct monitoring of thrombin generation by the splitting of chromogenic substrate. If thrombin generation is to be monitored a two stage setup remains necessary. Also in tests for prothrombin the activation has to take place without the chromogenic substrate being present i.e. a pre-incubation will be always necessary.

1.3. Antithrombin III and heparin cofactor

Various approaches have been published to measure antithrombin III c.q. heparin cofactor (10–18). Its inactivating action against both thrombin and factor X_a have been used. Here we summarise those methods employing thrombin. For other methods, see p. 104.

Usually citrated plasma is used in these tests. It may or may not be heat defibrinated (5 min at 53°C with immersion in ice after heating). This procedure is compulsory in methods based on the clotting of fibrinogen but it is often not necessary in chromogenic tests because of the high dilution of the sample and because of the chromogenic substrate inhibiting to some extent the action of thrombin on fibrinogen. The outcome of the test is influenced by the procedure however (18). Occasionally defibration by Arvin (snake venom) or by adsorbtion onto bentonite (ref) (snake venom) is attempted.

All methods for antithrombin III are bioassays, in the sense that quantification is obtained by comparison of the inactivation brought about by a (dilution of a) standard sample and of the unknown sample. The thrombin concentration used varies roughly between 0.1 and 1 NIHU per μl of undiluted plasma sample in the test. As to heparin there are two possibilities. Either there is heparin present in the sample in such a low concentration that it will not influence the test (e.g. < 1 U/ml of plasma in Bergströms setup) (12) and/or it is neutralised by polybrene (30 μg/ml will neutralise heparin up to 50 U/ml of heparin but does not adversely influence the test) (10) or an excess of heparin is added so as to potentiate maximally the antithrombin III present (8–10 U per μl of undiluted plasma present in the test).

In the tests of the first generation S 2160 is used at a concentration of about 0.1 mM, which equals K_m. Later S 2238 could be used high above K_m. Interesting is the use of a fluorogenic substrate (Cbz-Gly-Pro-Arg(HCC)-4 methoxy-β naphtylamide. Enzyme system products inc. Ind. U.S.A.) at a concentration of 0.23 mM is about $3 \times K_m$ (14).

A typical setup is the following. The sample is diluted 1/60 with a buffer containing heparin. (Tris/HCl 0.05 M, pH 8.4, EDTA 7.5 mM, heparin 3 U/ml, NaCl 0.075 M), 400 μl of this mixture plus 100 μl of thrombin (10–15 NIHU/ml) are incubated for 30 sec. Then 200 μl of a solution of 750 mM in S 2238 (or Chromosym TH) containing 0.3 mg/ml of polybene is added. Colour production can be measured kinetically or in an endpoint procedure if, after 30 sec exactly 600 μl of 50% acetic acid solution is added.

The standard error of the determination is about 5%. High correlation coefficients (r from 0.85 to 0.97) are found between the level of antithrombin III measured in this way and the levels assessed by immunochemical or clotting assays. The test may be influenced by high levels of bilirubin or highly lipaemic plasma when the end point method is used. When the final dilution of plasma is 1/60 bilirubin levels of < 5 μg/ml will not interfere.

1.4. Prothrombinase, factor V, platelet factor 3

S 2238 can be used conveniently to monitor the velocity of thrombin formation from a known amount of prothrombin and hence to assess the activity of the prothrombin splitting enzyme complex (prothrombinase). If factor X_a is present in a fixed concentration that is relatively high compared to the other components of the prothrombinase complex (e.g. by activating a sufficient amount of factor X with Russell's Viper Venom) then either in the presence of a fixed high concentration of factor V the amount of prothrombinase depends on the amount of suitable *phospholipid* present, or in the presence of a fixed amount of phospholipid, *factor V* can be the rate determining reaction constituant.

It should be remembered that S 2238 effectively inhibits factor X_a

both in the presence and the absence of phospholipids and factor V. Therefore the presence of the substrate in the activation mixture is better avoided.

Subsampling from the activation mixture at different time intervals and subsequent testing for the thrombin generated gives the best results. Alternatively testing after a fixed period of preincubation may be tried out.

In the literature there is some confusion as to the exact meaning of the term platelet factor 3. It can be thought to mean (a) lipid material obtained from platelets, (b) procoagulant lipid on the surface of the activated platelet, (c) procoagulant lipid as sub (b) plus factor V_a released by the platelet. In definition (a) the lipid material from lysed platelets is included, in definition (b) not. There is no way of differentiating between these two by means of a kinetic assay. Differentiation can be made by centrifugation or measurement of released enzymes (e.g., lactate dehydrogenase) but this subject is beyond the scope of this book.

1.4.1. Prothrombinase

It has been shown (19) that the action of the complete prothrombinase complex (i.e. factor X_a, factor V and phospholipid) on prothrombin obeys Michaelis Menten Kinetics, but also that the kinetic parameters are dependent upon the amount and composition of the lipid present. Typical values are V_{max}: 30–45 mole II. mole X_a^{-1}. sec^{-1}; K_m: 5×10^{-5} M to 2×10^{-3} M. The high value of K_m is found at $75 \mu M$ phospholipid (equal molar amounts of phosphatidyl serine and phosphatidyl choline). Such a mixture contains about $0.5 \mu M$ of binding sites for factor X_a and in this is equivalent to more than 10^{11} activated platelets/ml.

It can be assumed that in platelet rich plasma and in artificial mixtures the phospholipid concentration can be adjusted so as to provide no more than 5×10^{-8} M binding sites (about $7.5 \mu M$ of the most effective phospholipid). In that case $K_m \approx 0.1 \mu M$ which is well below the mean plasma concentration (about $1.5 \mu M$). It can be concluded that as a rule the normal plasma concentration of prothrombin will be well above the prevailing K_m of a complete prothrombinase. In that case at least 30 molecules of thrombin will be formed per molecule of prothrombinase per second. Due to the variations of V_{max} and K_m with the composition of the prothrombinase these data can only be used to get a rough estimate of the activities to be expected and not to calculate concentrations of prothrombinase. These are again better assessed by comparison to `standards, the nature of the standard depending upon the rate limiting component of prothrombinase that is to be determined. (See also (19)). The variation of the kinetic constants with the concentration of the constituents of the enzyme in fact precludes measuring prothrombinase activity by anything else than a bioassay. Even if it be a bioassay that uses the conversion of a chromogenic substrate as an indicator.

1.4.2. Factor V
Factor V can be measured in the following way: (personal communication T. Lindhout).

The factor V in the sample is first activated with Russel's Viper Venom (Stypven) ($100 \mu l$ sample is incubated with $5 \mu l$ Russel's Viper Venom (0.1 mg/ml) for 1 min at room temperature) and afterwards the following additions are made to the activation mixture:

Tris/HCl (50 mM, pH 7.4, 0.1 M NaCl) $400 \mu l$
phospholipid suspension (1 part Brain PS
and 3 parts egg PC, 50 mg/ml) $100 \mu l$
factor X_a preparation ($5 \times 10^{-5} \mu M$) $200 \mu l$
$CaCl_2$ (50 mM) $100 \mu l$

(All solutions are made in buffer as indicated)

After 5 min of incubation at $37°C$, $100 \mu l$ of a $10 \mu M$ solution of prothrombin is added. After exactly 2 min the reaction is stopped by pipetting 1 ml of a solution containing 0.4 mg/ml Soybean Trypsin Inhibitor and 0.47 mM S 2238 and the rate of colour production is measured. If necessary, ovalbumin may be added to the test system (final concentration 0.5 mg/ml). 10^{-14} Mole of factor V_a will cause an adsorbancy change of roughly 0.5 AU per min. $1 \mu l$ of normal plasma contains about 2×10^{-14} gMol of factor V. Normal plasma therefore should be diluted $1:10 000$ in this test.

1.4.3. Platelet factor 3 (20)
In platelet rich citrated plasma the platelets are first counted and then diluted with Hepes buffer to obtain a concentration of 5×10^6 platelets ml.$^{-1}$ (Composition of the buffer: Hepes: 10 mM, pH 7,4; NaCl: 137 mM; KCl: 2.68 mM; $MgCl_2$: 1.7 mM; glucose; 25 mM; fat free bovine serum albumin; 0.5 mg/ml).

To $250 \mu l$ of this suspension is added
   $50 \mu l$ $CaCl_2$ 30 mM in the same buffer
   $50 \mu l$ collagen suspension ($100 \mu g/ml$)
   $50 \mu l$ Thrombin (20 nM at $t = 0$)
exactly 8 min after the last addition is added:
   $50 \mu l$ factor X_a (5 nM)
and 2 min later (at $t = 10$)
   $50 \mu l$ factor II ($10 \mu M$)

The complete reaction is carried out at 37°C under continuous stirring. At $\frac{1}{2}$, 1 and $1\frac{1}{2}$ min after the last addition a subsample of 25 μl of the mixture is added to 1 ml of a buffer containing Tris/HCl 30 mM, pH 7,8; NaCl: 120 mM; EDTA: 2 mM. Then 1 ml of a 0.5 mM solution of S 2238 is added and the amount of thrombin in the sample is estimated from comparison of the velocity measured with that obtained with a standard preparation of thrombin. From the three different subsamples the rate of thrombin formation can be calculated. The values obtained are in the order of magnitude of 10 nM of thrombin formed per minute.

The assay records platelet prothrombin converting activity which consists of two components: release and activation of factor V and generation of binding sites for the prothrombin complex.

To make the assay sensitive to the binding sites only an excess of factor V_a can be added, e.q. by including 5 nM F.V_a in the factor X_a solution.

IV.2. Factor X_a and derived determinations

Factor X_a can be readily measured with two chromogenic substrates, S2222 and S2337. There exist two distinct forms of factor X called factor X_1 and factor X_2. The difference may reside in the esterification of a side chain (21) no difference in function or activity between these forms have been observed either for the activated or the unactivated molecule. From one form of factor X, two forms of factor X_a can be made, called $FX_a\alpha$ and $FX_a\beta$ (22). Most kinetic properties have probably been determined in preparations rich in (c.q. consisting of) Factor X_ab. There are no indications that the kinetic properties of the α and the β form towards synthetic substrates are different (23).

2.1. Factor X_a

A practical setup for the measurement of factor X_a is the following:

Medium: Tris HCl pH 7,8 : 50 mM
          NaCl   : 175 mM

If purified Factor X_a is to be determined, ovalbumin (0.5 mg/ml) will prevent the denaturation occuring in very dilute solutions. If further activation of factor ·X is to be stopped e.g. when subsampling from a factor X activating mixture, EDTA to a concentration of 10 mM may be added. *Substrate*: one tenth of the final volume of a solution of 3.3 mg/ml of S 2222 is added so as to obtain a final concentration of 0.45 mM which approximately equals K_m. For S 2337 this is about the same.

In this experimental setup the rate of initial colour production at 405 nm will be about 0.043 AU per min per nM X_a (at 37°C).

Factor X_a in intact plasma can be measured if the plasma (blood) immediately upon venapuncture is mixed with an excess of anti-antithrombin III immunoglobin (24). This lengthens the survival time of factor X_a, without abolishing factor X_a inactivation altogether, possibly because of the presence of protease inhibitors other than antithrombin III or α_2-macroglobin (whose action will hardly be observed because the α_2-M factor X_a complex still splits small substrates). This test has been carried out with a plasma dilution of about 7 x (depending upon hematocrit) in a medium of isotonic Tris/HCl buffer pH 8.4, with S 2222 at 0.250 mM as a substrate.

The abnormal factor X_a then can arise from activation of decarboxy factor X (PIVKA-X) by the action of Russell Viper Venom (23) has the same kinetic properties towards S 2222 as the normal factor has.

The estimation of factor X_a can serve as the basis for the assessment of factor X, antithrombin III (and thus heparin and platelet factor 4) and the constituents of the factor X activating enzymes i.e. Factor VII, Factor VIII, Factor IX, phospholipid (platelet factor 3) and tissue thromboplastin. Several of the possible tests have been worked out. Ameliorations of some of the tests are still to be expected as many of them are 'first generation' anyhow.

2.2. Factor X

For the determination of factor X in plasma the factor X activating protease from Russells Viper Venom (RVV-X) seems to be the activator of choice. No lipid is necessary in this reaction. In fact lipid inhibits because RVV-X acts only on free, non adsorbed factor X (25). In the absence of lipid negligible amounts of thrombin are formed. Thus a possible source of error is excluded. If thromboplastin and factor VII are used as an activator also less factor X_a seems to form than with RVV-X. With thromboplastin as an activator the amount of factor X_a formed is only linear with the amount of plasma in standard samples over a short range of concentrations and the coefficient of variation is larger than with the RVV-X method (26). Of the published manual methods (26, 6) a typical example follows:

Buffer (Tris HCl 50 mM pH 8.3; 0.10 M NaCl)   0.410 ml
Citrated plasma   0.015 ml
Russells Viper Venom solution (0.12‰ w/v in buffer)   0.050 ml

CaCl$_2$ (0.5 M)	0.025 ml
Incubation at 37°C for 60 sec	
S 2222 (1 mM)	2.000 ml

The velocity of substrate conversion is followed continuously in a spectrophotometer. Automatised factor X determinations have been described and seem to be practically feasible (27, 28). A commercialized test kit for Factor X estimation is available (Kabivitrium Coatest®/Factor X).

RVV-X will activate decarboxy factor X but does this only slowly (23). This activation apparently does not influence the tests results (27).

2.3 Antifactor X_a (antithrombin III, heparin cofactor)

The major part of total antifactor X_a measured in plasma consists of antithrombin III (At III). The other important factor X_a antagonist is α_2 Macroglobin (α_2 M) but the α_2 M-factor X_a complex retains its amidolytic activity towards chromogenic substrates and thus does not contribute to any significant extent to the inactivation observed in spectrophotometric assays.

In the presence of heparin the affinity of antithrombin III for factor X_a is much larger than in its absence. In kinetic tests for antithrombin III, all antithrombin III should either react quickly or slowly, so the test should be carried out either in complete absence of heparin or in the presence of an excess of heparin. In the absence of heparin, plasma protease inhibitors other than antithrombin III will account for a relatively large part of the velocity of factor X_a disappearance (around 20%); in the presence of heparin their contribution will be hardly noticed. A typical assay may be run as follows (29);

Plasma diluted 1:200 in buffer*	0.200 ml
Factor X_a in buffer (4 U/ml; 75 pM)	0.100 ml
incubate 30 sec	
S 2222 (1 mM, polybrene 0.3 mg/ml)	0.200 ml
incubate 420 sec	
acetic acid (50%)	0.300 ml

*buffer: 50 mM Tris/HCl. pH 8.4, I = 0.21, containing EDTA 75 mM and heparin 3 U/ml.

The results are read against a standard curve made with 1/800–1/150 dilutions of normal plasma. In this test heparin is present during the inactivation of factor X_a and neutralised only during the measurement of residual amidolytic acitivity. Alternatively a 1/10 dilution of plasma in a buffer containing 50 μg/ml of polybrene can be used. In that case the first incubation should last 300 sec and the standard curve is made with 1/40 to 1/6 diluted normal plasma. A slightly different setup is published by Mattler (30). The authors make the following observations:

1. Defibrination is not necessary and does not significantly influence the results. Neither do fibrinogen degradation products.
2. If all antithrombin III is removed from a sample by immunoabsorbtion then hardly any activity remains if the first variant, i.e. that including heparin, is used. When no heparin is present in the test, after removal of antithrombin III there is a persistant factor X_a inactivating potential of about 20% of the original, due to inactivators other than antithrombin III or α_2 M.
3. Standard deviation in duplicate analysis is about 4.5%. This compares well to the coagulation method (9%).
4. There is a strong positive correlation between this test and the results of a conventional heparin cofactor assay ($R = 0.85$). The second variant shows less correlation ($R = 0.58$).

The method can be readily automated (31). There are commercialized kits available also (Coatest Kabivitrum®, Antithrombin III Boehringer).

2.4. Heparin

If antithrombin III is present in excess over heparin, the amount of heparing-antithrombin III complex and hence the amount of heparin will determine the rate of rapid inactivation of factor X_a. In this way heparin can be estimated in essentially the same setup as the antithrombin III test described above. A typical procedure is (32):

plasma	0.100 ml
Antithrombin III (1 U/ml; $\approx$ 2 nM)	0.100 ml
Buffer (Tris/HCl pH 8.4, 50 mM; NaCl 0.175 M; EDTA 7.5 mM)	0.800 ml
An aliquot of this mixture of 0.200 ml is added to factor X_a (bovine) (8 U/ml; 150 pM)	0.100 ml
and incubated for 180 (or 30) sec, then S 2222 (1 mM)	0.200 ml
is incubated for 240 (or 120) sec, and the reaction stopped with acetic acid (50%)	0.300 ml

The incubation times in brackets are used to assess high concentrations of heparin: 0.04–0.80 U/ml. The other incubation times are suitable with low heparin concentrations: 0.01–0.20 U/ml. Instead of a purified preparation, pooled normal plasma can be used as a source of antithrombin III. This has the theoretical disadvantage of adding possible heparin independent factor X_a inactivators or heparin binding substances.

This will not interfere to any significant extent when heparin levels are above 0.02 U/ml.

A linear relation between absorbancy and heparin concentration is reported to be obtained up till 0.6 U/ml of heparin (resp. 0.15 U/ml in the setup for low concentrations). A bilirubin level of more than $60 \mu g/ml$ plasma will influence the readings unless individual blanks are used. In the therapeutic range (0.2–0.7 U/ml) the coefficient of variation of this method is around 9%, which compares favourable to clotting assays. In the low ranges the accuracy rapidly diminished. For a further discussion see Teien (32) and van Putten (34).

In heparin estimations the sampling technique and storage of blood may be important. Platelet rich plasma in which the platelets are activated or lysed cause heparin activity to diminish progressively. Blood should be kept on ice until centrifuged for 20 min at 2.000 g (4°C). If further storage is necessary the plasma is preferably first spun platelet free (up to 30 min at 12.000 g, 4°C). Platelet counts below $15\,000/\mu l$ will not influence the test to any appreciable extent. A commercialized form of the test is available (Coatest®/heparin Kabivitrum) that seems to do fairly well in monitoring heparin treatment (33). Still heparin determination is not a solved problem.

A comparative study of heparin estimations (34) shows that
a. thrombin times and whole blood recalcification time do *not* allow heparin quantitation.
b. activated partial thromboplastin time (APTT) with heparin titration allows a semiquantitative determination of heparin levels.
c. Amidolytic methods are the best tests available but only if it is recognised that the reference line is not linear.
d. No methods are available to assess plasma heparin levels below 0.2 U/ml.

2.5. Platelet factor 4 and other antiheparins

Plasma as well as platelets contain a number of heparin binding substances. Platelet factor 4 (Pf 4) is a protein form platelets that specifically binds heparin. It is liberated during the release reaction of platelets. The antiheparin activity in platelet free plasma (c.q. plasma with unstimulated platelets) can be used as an estimate of the non Pf 4 antiheparins. The crux of this approach is in obtaining plasma without activating platelets.

Bolton *et al.* (35) using plasma collected in a cocktail containing EDTA, theophylline and Prostaglandin E, showed that much Pf 4 previously thought to be present in normal plasma actually is derived from platelets activated after venapuncture during the processing of the plasma. Normal plasma concentrations are below $10 \mu g/l$ (35). The main plasma anti-heparin activity is probably α_1-acid glycoprotein one of the acute phase proteins. (37).

In order to estimate the contribution of Pf 4 to antiheparin activity in the plasma of a patient one has to carry out three determinations (38). First one eliminates the Pf 4 present by adding an anti Pf 4 antibody to the sample. Then one maximally activates the platelets with epinephrin or collagen. Comparison of the untreated sample with these data makes it possible to estimate the contribution of free Pf 4 to the spontaneous antiheparin activity of the sample.

A typical setup is (39, 40)

sample (1:2 diluted plasma or platelet suspension containing 3×10^5 platelets)	0.100 ml
Antithrombin III (3.3 U/ml)	0.050 ml
Heparin (0.4 U/ml in distilled water)	0.050 ml
Factor X_a (5 U/ml)	0.100 ml
Incubation for 60 sec.	
S 2222 (2 mM in 2 mM Tris/HCl pH 8.4 NaCl 0.15 M).	0.250 ml

Endpoint measurements can be made if the reaction is stopped after 60 sec with 0.300 ml of 50% acetic acid.

2.6. Factor X activating enzymes

There are two physiological factor X activating enzymes. The 'intrinsic' one consisting of factor IX_a, factor VIII_a and phospholipid and the 'extrinsic' one consisting of factor VII_a and thromboplastin. Although the sharp distinction between the extrinsic and the intrinsic pathway is fading in the light of recent research we will still use these designations for the two types of factor X activator. The intrinsic activator has been studied extensively by van Dieijen et al. (41), the extrinsic one by the group of Nemerson (42).

The complete intrinsic enzyme, that consists of factor IX_a, factor VIII_a and phospholipid has a K_m for factor X of $0.06-1.80 \mu M$ and a V_{max} of $2.50-4.40$ Mole $X_a \cdot min^{-1} \cdot$ Mole IX_a^{-1}. The large variation is due to the fact that the apparent K_m and V_{max} both are dependent upon the phospholipid concentrations. This, together with the fact that factor VIII cannot be added in saturating amounts shows clearly that rigorous standardisation is a prerequisite for the determination of individual components of the tenase complex. Even in this way it will be hardly possible to estimate the concentration of a rate limiting component of the tenase complex (be it phospholipid, factor VIII of factor IX) from the observed turnover of factor X and knowledge of the kinetic constants.

It therefore remains necessary to use standard preparations in order to make reference curves and the methods remain essentially bio-assays. Still their accuracy and the possibility of automation make them interesting alternatives for the usual clotting assay.

2.6.1. Factor VIII
In 1978 a method for factor VIII determination has been published (43). An investigation into its usefulness in the practice of treating hemofiliacs and screening for (acquired) inhibitors is as yet lacking. We have no personal experience with this method.

2.6.2. Factor IX
The method reported here is described in refs. (44) and (45). The method is carried out in a medium consisting of Tris-HCl 50 mM, pH 7.9 at 22°C, NaCl 175 mM. For this method a factor XI_a preparation is necessary that is prepared from bovine plasma according to Østerund and Rapaport (46) and solved in buffer to a concentration of 1.5 mg/ml. Brain phosphatidylserine and egg phosphatidylcholine in a 1:3 ratio are suspended by sonication to a final concentration of 1 mM. Factor X is purified as described by Fujikawa et al. (47) and kept in a stock solution of 0.55 mg/ml.

The determination runs as follows:

Between 5 and 40 μl of the sample plasma are incubated with 1.5 μg of factor XI_a in a final volume of 1 ml buffer (which is made 10 mM in $CaCl_2$ and 0.5 mg/ml in ovalbumin) for 25 min at 37°C.

0.1 ml of this mixture is added to 0.25 ml buffer, containing 0.5 mg/ml of ovalbumin, 0.05 ml factor X solution, 0.05 ml of phospholipid suspension and 0.05 ml of $CaCl_2$ 0.1 M. After 10 min at 37°C, 0.4 ml of the mixture is added to a cuvet that contains 1.5 ml buffer with 0.5 mg/ml ovalbumin and 20 mM EDTA, then 0.1 ml of S 2222 (3.86 mM) is added and the adsorbancy change recorded.

2.6.3. Platelet factor 3
Up to this moment the phospholipid component of the tenase complex as present in the intact triggered platelet has been determined spectrophotometrically only in experiments designed to investigate the mechanism of platelet activation (20) no routine determinations in patients have been carried out. The method of Sandberg and Andersson (48) measures the combined effect of platelet lysis and activation.

2.6.4. Factor VII and tissue thromboplastin
In principle both factor VII and tissue thromboplastins can be tested through their activating actions on factor X. In this field several difficulties

arise that at this moment have not been solved. Useful methods for factor VII determinations have been published (49, 50). They determine total Factor VII on basis of a complete activation of this factor. The problems arise from the fact that factor VII is present in plasma in two species, the one chain and the two chains form. The former one has a distinct species specificity whereas the latter one has not (51). Also the two chain form does arise in certain plasmas upon storage in the cold, whereas it also has been suggested that the two chain form is indicative of different forms of disease such as metastases from carcinoma of the prostrate and generalised atherosclerosis. As yet there are no methods available to differentiate between the two forms in a chromogenic assay only. On the other hand, if tissue thromboplastins of different species have to be compared the result of a test will differ depending on the relative amount of the two chain form of Factor VII present in the test. This greatly hampers standardisation in this type of test.

A further complication may result from the fact that factor X_a will activate Factor VII.

The effect of a chromogenic substrate occupying Factor X_a active sites on the interaction with Factor VII remains to be investigated.

Determination of Factor VII

human plasma (diluted between 1:80 and 1:400)	0.100 ml
Tissue thromboplastin (human brain)	0.050 ml
Factor X solution (1.8 U/ml in buffer)	0.050 ml
Incubation in a plastic tube at 37°C for 1 min	
CaCl$_2$ 50 mM (prewarmed)	0.025 ml
Incubation for 3 min at 37°C	
0.3 M Na$_2$ EDTA	
the tube is placed on ice and a 0.1 ml subsample is transferred to a cuvette containing	
S 2222 (1 mg/ml)	0.100 ml
Tris/HCl (50 mM, pH 7.5, NaCl 0.15 M)	0.600 ml

The velocity of colour production at 405 mM is recorded and compared to the velocity obtained with different dilutions of a standard plasma.

IV.3. Determination of fibrinolytic pathway components in plasma (53, 54, 56) (Contributed by K.C. Robbins and R.C. Wohl)

3.1. Plasminogen

Two chromogenic substrates have been used for measuring plasminogen concentration, both methods giving the same results. A $20\,\mu$l sample of plasma and a 40 μl sample of streptokinase (50.000 IU/ml) (9 M excess of streptokinase to plasminogen) were mixed in a test tube and incubated at 37°C. At the end of 15 min, a 30 μl sample was withdrawn and added to a semimicrocuvette in a Beckman 25 Spectrophotometer. In the esterase assay method, the cuvette contained 920 μl of 0.1 M sodium phosphate/0.1 M NaCl buffer, pH 6.0 and 50 μl of 4.5×10^{-3} M Nα-Cbz-L-lysine-p-nitrophenyl ester at 37°C. The rate of spontaneous hydrolysis of the ester substrate in the buffer is established by addition of the substrate to the buffer two minutes prior to addition of the plasma-streptokinase aliquot. The spontaneous substrate hydrolysis was subtracted from the initial velocity, or net absorbance change per min. A velocity of $v = 0.186 A_{340}$ per min was equivalent to 20.0 mg plasminogen/dl plasma using a standard curve, up to 40 mg plasminogen/dl plasma, prepared with pure Glu-plasminogen. When the tripeptide amide substrate, H-D-Val-Leu-Lys-pNA, was used, the cuvette contained 960 μl of 0.05 M Tris/0.1 M NaCl buffer, pH 7.4, and 10 μl of 1×10^{-2} M substrate at 37°C. A velocity of $v = 0.125 A_{405}$ per min is equivalent to 20.0 mg plasminogen/dl plasma. Normal range: 16.7–23.8 mg/dl; mean of 20.25 mg/dl with a standard deviation of 2.24 mg/dl.

3.2 Plasminogen activator

A semimicro cuvette containing 415 μl of 0.05 M Tris/0.1 M NaCl buffer, pH 7.4, was warmed to 37°C. Twenty-five μl of 1×10^{-2} M H-D-Val-Leu-Lys-pNA solution and 10 μl Lys-plasminogen (25 μg), completely activatable, are added and a baseline established at 405 nM. After 2 to 3 min, 50 μl of plasma is added and the reaction is followed until an absorbance change of between 0.5 to 1.0 A is obtained. The net absorbance change divided by time increments ($\Delta A/t$) is plotted against the time increment values (t), and a straight line is drawn. The slope of this line is equivalent to $b/2$; b is proportional to the initial velocity of plasminogen activation. A value of b equivalent to 0.066 per min^2 is equal to 25.0 IU streptokinase activity/ml of plasma, or 84.2 IU urokinase activity/ml of plasma. These activator activity concentration values are based on the kinetic constants previously described (55) for plasminogen activation by streptokinase and urokinase. Plasminogen activator concentrations as low as 0.01 IU/ml of plasma can be measured by this method. Normal: no detectable activity.

3.3. 'Free' protease activity

A 500 μl plasma sample is introduced into a semimicrocuvette, warmed to 37°C, and 25 μl of 1×10^{-2} M H-D-Val-Leu-Lys-pNA solution is added. The initial velocity, or net absorbance change per min, of hydrolysis is followed for about 5 min, and then 5 KIU of Trasylol are added. The inhibited portion of the hydrolytic activity is considered 'free' protease activity and can be converted into 'free' plasmin activity. A velocity of $1.0 A_{405}$ per min (1.0×10^{-4} per min p-nitroaniline formed) is equal to 0.74 mg plasmin/dl plasma. This factor is calculated from the kinetic parameters of plasmin for the peptide substrate. Normal: no detectable activity.

3.4. Plasmin generation rates

Twenty-five μl of 1×10^{-2} M H-D-Val-Leu-Lys-pNA solution are added to a 500 μl plasma sample in a semimicrocuvette at 37°C; after 3 min, 10 μl of either urokinase (containing 250 IU) or streptokinase (containing 25 IU) are added (system at pH 7.4). After 3 min of activation, the net absorbance change at 405 nm, after subtraction of amidase activity before addition of activator, is multiplied by a factor of 0.735 for urokinase or by a factor of 15.934 for streptokinase to obtain % observable velocity. This is the calculated initial velocity of plasminogen activation in plasma (v_{obs}) divided by the calculated initial velocity generated in a pure plasminogen solution ($v_{calc.}$), under the same conditions. The conversion factors are derived from kinetic parameters. The net change in absorbance indicates plasminogen activation only if the absorbance change accelerates with time.

Normal range: (a) urokinase: 0.25–0.47% observable velocity; mean of 0.37% with a standard deviation of 0.13%.

(b) streptokinase: 5.30–9.70% observable velocity, mean of 7.02% with a standard deviation of 1.67%.

3.5. α_2-Plasmin inhibitor

The measurement of the initial velocity of hydrolysis of 1×10^{-4} M H-D-Val-Leu-Lys-pNA, in 1.0 ml of 0.05 M Tris/0.1 M NaCl buffer, pH 7.4, by 4.0 μg plasmin (30 IU/mg protein) at 37°C, at 405 nm, is carried out. A solution containing 200 μg plasmin/ml (stock solution in a pH 7.4 buffer containing 25% glycerol) was used. The inhibitor assay is performed by the addition of 20 μl of plasma to 950 μl of the above buffer in a semimicro cuvette at 37°C, followed by the addition of 20 μl of plasmin (4.0 μg plasmin). Ten μl of 1×10^{-2} M H-D-Val-Leu-Lys-pNA solution is added 20 sec after the addition of the plasmin, and the initial velocity, or net absorbance change per min, is measured. To convert the percent plasmin inhibited data to concentration of α_2-plasmin inhibitor, the fraction of plasmin inhibited is multiplied by a factor of 0.16 which

Table IV.2.   Units of urokinase

1.	IU = 0.70 Ploug U = 1.03 CTA
1.	CTA = 0.68 Ploug U = 0.97 IU
1. Ploug U. = 1.43 IU = 1.48 CTA
1. IU High Mol. Weight Urokinase is about 1.8×10^{-11} Mole
1. IU Low Mol. Weight Urokinase is about 1.4×10^{-11} Mole

is equal to $0.2 \times$ mol.wt. α_2-plasmin inhibitor/mol.wt.plasmin. The factor converts μg plasmin inhibited per $20\,\mu l$ of plasma to mg α_2-plasmin inhibitor/dl plasma. Normal range: 6.4–8.0 mg/dl.

IV.4. The contact activation system

4.1. Plasma prekallikrein

Plasma prekallikrein (PPK), previously also known under the name of Fletcher factor in coagulation literature, can be activated to yield plasma kallikrein (PK) that is active upon the artificial substrate S 2302.

Factor XII, plasma prekallikrein and high molecular weight kinnogen (HMWK) interact in a complicated fashion when blood comes into contact with wettable surfaces or certain other activators. For an extensive review of these reactions the reader is referred to the literature (57). Summarising very briefly one can say that F XII and PPK mutually activate each other if a suitable surface (or a substance like ellagic acid) and HMWK are present.

Activated factor XII can activate factor XI. The contact system also activates plasminogen. In congenital deficiences of factor XII (Hageman deficiency) PPK (Fletcher deficiency) or HMWK (Fleaujac, Fitzgerald or Williams trait) no proper generation of S 2303 converting activity can be expected. By manipulating the system so that one of these factors becomes rate limiting, it can be made into a test system for that factor. This has been worked out for PPK (58, 59, 60, 61, 62, 63) and for factor XII (62) but not as yet for HMWK.

Plasma prekallikrein determination (58)
    The following set up does work in practice:

Plasma in suitable dilution (1/4–1/30)	0.100 ml
Tris/Imidazole buffer pH 7.8, 50 mM, I 0.05 (NaCl)	1.500 ml
Activator	0.700 ml
Incubation for 3 min at 37°C	
Substrate solution	0.200 ml

Record OD change continuously or stop the reaction at 3 min (with 1 ml 50% acetic acid) to obtain an endpoint measurement.

The choice of the most suitable activator seems not to be settled as yet. In the above example a 1:10 dilution of Cephotest (Nygaard) has been used, but also kaolin (1% w/v) in buffer or dextran sulphate (MW 500.000, 25 mg/ml) can be employed (64). Also the use as an activator of a celite eluate, rich in factor XII and HMWK but poor in kallikrein (prep. acc. to Ogston e.a. 65) has been described (63).

The reference curves are always obtained with dilutions of normal plasma as the source of the rate limiting factor. Usually it is quoted that the assay is independent of factor XII and probably HMWK if these proteins are present above a certain minimal percentage (25–40%). Also the amount of PK formed can be dependent upon the amount as well as upon the batch of activator used (61). At substrate concentration higher than 1.47 mM a strong inhibition by the substrate chromozym PK has been observed.

A maximum of 4% of the total activity observed in this system could be attributed to plasmin. Factor X_a formation will not interfere. Epsilonaminocaproic acid (1 mg/ml final concentration) has been used to suppress the action of plasmin (62). The coefficient of variation of this test was found to be between 2 and 8%.

Fluorogenic plasma prekallikrein determination (66)
(Contributed by S. Iwanaga, H. Kato, T. Morita, T. Sugo, Y. Ohno, M. Ohki, K. Takada, S. Sakakibara)
Principle: Prekallikrein in human plasma is activated with acetone and kaolin, and the enzyme activity evolved is measured using the fluorescence of carbobenzoxy (Z)-Phe-Arg-MCA as the substrate.
Reagents:
Human plasma: The plasma is collected into plastic tubes containing 1/10 volume of 3.8% sodium citrate.
Kaolin: Kaolin (K-5) from Fisher Scientific Co., Pittsburgh, Pennsylvania.
Trypsin inhibitors: Soybean and Lima bean trypsin inhibitors (Worthington Biochem. Co., Freehold, New Jersey.)
Buffer I: 0.02 M Tris/HCl, pH 8.0, containing 0.15 M NaCl.
Buffer II: 0.05 M Tris/HCl, pH 8.0, containing 0.1 M NaCl and 0.01 M $CaCl_2$.
Substrate: Z-Phe-Arg-MCA is dissolved at 1×10^{-2} M in dimethyl-sulfoxide (stock solution) and diluted to 5×10^{-5} M in Buffer II just prior to the assay.
Procedure: Citrated human plasma (50 μl) is mixed with 850 μl of a solution consisting of 700 μl Buffer I and 150 μl acetone) and allowed to stand for 10 min at room temperature (25°C). Then 100 μl Kaolin

suspension (10 mg/ml of Buffer I) is added and mixed vigorously using an electric mixer for 15 sec. At certain time intervals after the addition of Kaolin, 20 μl aliquots of the above mixture are taken and transferred into 1 ml of 5×10^{-5} M Z-Phe-Arg-MCA solution containing either 40 μg of lima bean trypsin inhibitor (tube A) or 40 μg of soybean trypsin inhibitor (tube B). After incubation for 10 min at 37°C, the reaction is terminated by the addition of 2 ml of 17% acetic acid, and the fluorescence read at 460 nm (emission) and 380 nm (excitation) in a Hitachi MPF-3 fluorescence spectrophotometer. The difference between the values from tube A and tube B is calculated as prekallikrein activity. One unit of prekallikrein is arbitrary defined as the amount of enzyme which releases 1×10^{-7} M AMC/10 min under the described conditions.

Comments: The kallikrein generated under above conditions is stable for 60 min after activation and at least 10% of the original concentration of both Hageman factor and high molecular weight kininogen are required to obtain complete activation of prekallikrein within this time period. When Fletcher trait plasma is assayed for prekallikrein, it shows no detectable activity. When this plasma is mixed with varying proportions of normal plasma, the prekallikrein content of the normal plasma can readily be detected. The lower concentrations of normal plasma activate more slowly but all dilutions reach a maximum in 60 min. When the data at 60 min are replotted, a linear relationship is obtained between the content of prekallikrein and hydrolysis of Z-Phe-Arg-MCA. Normal human plasma heated at 60°C for 60 min, forms no prekallikrein, and mixtures of this heated plasma with normal plasma forms kallikrein at levels that are proportional to the content of prekallikrein in the sample. When this method is compared to a radiochemical method employing ^{3}H-TAME (67) the sensitivity appears to be similar. Plasmin and hog pancreatic kallikrein less readily hydrolyze Z-Phe-Arg-MCA.

4.2. Factor XII

The principle of the estimation of factor XII(a) is the same as that for prekallikrein, the reaction conditions being selected so that in this case factor XII is the rate determining factor. The test was carried out as follows (62) 500 μl of plasma is incubated with a 500 μl of a $\frac{1}{2}$% (w/v) kaolin suspension in Tris (50 mM) buffered isotonic saline (pH 7.4). After 3 min incubation at 37°C the kaolin is centrifuged off at 2000 × g for 10 min. Then the sample is incubated at 37°C for 60 min which inactivates the kallikrein formed but not (or considerably less) the factor XII$_a$. Then normal nonactivated plasma is added (as a source of prekallikrein) as well as epsilonaminocaproic acid (EACA) (so as to inhibit plasmin) according to the following scheme:

Kaolin activated test plasma	0.100 ml
normal non activated plasma	0.050 ml
EACA (10 mg/ml)	0.050 ml
after 60 sec of incubation:	
S 2302 (0.67 mM) in 33 mM Tris/HCl pH 7.4	0.300 ml

The absorbancy change (ΔA) per minute was recorded at 405 nm.

It is remarked that
– between 1 and 100% linear calibration curves were obtained of initial ΔA/min versus the concentration of factor XII.
– The variation coefficient is about 8% as compared to 12% in a coagulation system.
– Kaolin is the activator of choice as it can be removed and thus will not in itself cause kallikrein formation from the non-activated normal plasma added afterwards.

Concluding remark
The mutual dependent activation of factor XII and prekallikrein at a wettable surface in the presence of high molecular weight kininogen (HMWK) as an accessory factor is a highly complicated biochemical mechanism the kinetics of which are still largely unknown. The use of the kallikrein substrates S 2302 and Chromozym PK undoubtedly allows to probe in directly into the contact phase of blood coagulation. Yet the precise conditions under which accurate quantification of any of the factors involved is reproducibly possible seems not to have been solved, because the dependency of the various tests on the level of the factors meant to be present in excess is not clear in all cases.

Fluorogenic assay method for activated factor XII (68)
(Contributed by S. Iwanaga, H. Kato, T. Morita, T. Sugo, Y. Ohno, M. Ohki, K. Takada, S. Sakakibara)

Principle: Among 36 peptidyl-MCA's so far synthesized, one substrate, Boc-Glu(OBz)-Gly-Arg-MCA, is most susceptible to splitting by Factor XII_a. Thus, the enzyme acticity is assayed on the basis of its amidase activity toward the substrate, using a fluorometer to estimate the amount of AMC released with time.

Reagents:

Factor XII_a: Bovine factor XII_a is purified according to the method of Fujikawa *et al.* (69). The protein concentration is determined from the absorbance at 280 nm using E_{280}^{1cm} value of 14.2 (69).

Buffer: 0.02 M Tris/HCl, pH 8.0, containing 0.15 M NaCl and bovine serum albumin (0.1 mg/ml).

Substrate: Boc-Glu(OBz)-Gly-Arg-MCA is dissolved in dimethylformamide, to give a final concentration of 10 mM.

Procedure: The mixture of 5 μl of the substrate and 500 μl of buffer is preincubated for 5 min in a 1.0 ml cuvette thermostated at 37°C. Then, 10 μl of Factor XII$_a$ ($A_{280} = 0.01$) is added and the increase of the relative fluorescence is read at regular time intervals (Initial-rate method).

Comments: Since the assay method described above is simple to perform, it is available for the quantitative estimation of factor XII$_a$ activity in the fraction obtained at the later stages of purification procedure. With Boc-Glu-(OBz)-Gly-Arg-MCA, Factor XII$_a$ activity is measured up to the factor XII$_a$ concentration of 0.1 μg per ml, and the rate of hydrolysis is proportional to enzyme concentration over at least a ten-fold range. Although the substrate is slightly hydrolyzed by plasma kallikrein, a specific assay of factor XII$_a$ can be obtained in the presence of pancreatic basic trypsin inhibitor (Trasylol®), because the kallikrein activity can be completely inhibited by the inhibitor without any effect on factor XII$_a$ activity. The use of this substance is also recommendable to estimate the amount of factor XII following its activation with plasma kallikrein (68).

4.3. Activated factor XI (70)
(Contributed by S. Iwanaga, H. Kato, T. Morita, T. Sugo, Y. Ohno, M. Ohki, K. Takada, S. Sakakibara)

Principle: A substrate, Boc-Phe-Ser-Arg-MCA, which is most susceptible to factor XI$_a$, is used and the amidase activity is measured fluorometrically.

Reagents:

Factor XI$_a$: Bovine factor XI is purified by the method of Koide et al. (71) and is activated by trypsin or factor XII$_a$, (10 μl factor XI solution (500 μg/ml), 600 μl Tris/HCl (0.02 M, pH 8.0, containing 0.15 M NaCl and 0.1 mg/ml bovine serum albumin) and 20 μl factor XII$_a$ (0.078 mg/ml) are incubated for 30 min at 37°C.) The protein concentration is determined from the absorbance at 280 nm using an $E_{280}^{1\,cm}$ value of 12.6 (80).

Buffer: 0.05 M Tris/HCl, pH 8.0, containing 0.15 M NaCl and bovine serum albumin (0.1 mg/ml).

Substrate: Boc-Phe-Ser-Arg-MCA is dissolved in dimethylformamide to give a final concentration of 10 mM.

Procedure: The mixture of 500 μl of buffer and 10 μl of factor XI$_a$ (about 10 μg protein) is preincubated for 5 min in a 1.0 ml cuvette thermostated at 37°C. Then, 5 μl of the substrate is rapidly admixed, and the initial rate of the increase of the relative fluorescence is read at regular time intervals.

Comments: Boc-Phe-Ser-Arg-MCA is a suitable substrate for factor XI_a estimation and the hydrolysis rate is constant over a long period up to 10 min. The proportionality between the amount of enzyme used and the activity measured is observed over a ten-fold range. Inactivation effects due to glass adsorption is minimal. Using this substrate, factor XI_a activity is quantitatively measured under the conditions described above up to a factor XI_a concentration of 0.5 μg/ml. Moreover, the sensitivity of the fluorescence due to AMC released can be amplified 10 times with the fluorimeter used, thus the limit of detection of factor XI_a by the initial-rate method is 50 ng/ml. The substrate Boc-Phe-Ser-Arg-MCA is very susceptible to trypsin. Therefore, soybean trypsin inhibitor should be added to the reaction mixture, if trypsin can be expected to be present in the sample. The use of this substrate is also recommendable to estimate the amount of factor XI following its activation with factor XII_a (70).

IV.5. Miscellaneous determinations

5.1. Glandular kallikrein

The method as published by Claesson (58) runs as follows:

Enzyme preparation	0.050 ml
Tris HCl (50 mM, pH 9.2 I = 0.05)	0.250 ml
Substrate (S 2266, 2 mM in water)	0.200 ml
The test is run at 37°C.	

Colour production can either be read continuously, or the reaction can be allowed to proceed for 4 min after which the reaction is stopped by adding 0.3 ml of concentrated acetic acid. Readings of about 80 ΔA/min per nkat/ml of enzyme, or 4.75 ΔA/min per U of enzyme are found. The coefficient of variation was found to be about 3%. The substrate is relatively insensitive towards urokinase.

Measurement for kallikrein in urine (72)
(Contributed by S. Iwanaga, H. Kato, T. Morita, T. Sugo, Y. Ohno, M. Ohki, K. Takada, S. Sakakibara)
Principle: Urinary kallikrein hydrolyzes specifically Pro-Phe-Arg-MCA, which is also good substrate for tissue kallikreins, and the product (AMC) after hydrolysis can be quantitated fluorometrically.

Reagents:

Human urine: A pooled urine is collected for 24 h.

Buffer: 0.1 M Tris/HCl, pH 8.0, containing 0.15 M NaCl.

Substrate: Pro-Phe-Arg-MCA is dissolved at 10 mM in dimethylform-amide.

Inhibitors: Bovine pancreatic trypsin inhibitor, Trasylol®, (Bayer Co., Germany) is dissolved in buffer (5,000 units/ml). 10% acetic acid.

Procedure: In 0.5 ml of 0.1 M Tris/HCl, pH 8.0, containing 0.15 M NaCl, 20 μl of urine and 5 μl of 10 mM Pro-Phe-Arg-MCA are added. After incubation for 90 min at 37°C, the reaction is terminated by adding 50 units of Trasylol® or 20 μl of 10% acetic acid. The amount of AMC liberated is measured using a Hitachi fluoroscence spectrophotometer, model MPF-2A. With excitation at 380 nm and emission at 440 nm. Kallikarin activity is expressed in terms of nmoles of AMC liberated per min.

Comments: Under the conditions described, the release of AMC increases linearly with incubation time up to 90 min. However, when the reaction rate is plotted against the amounts of urine, it does not increase linearly. The hydrolysis of Pro-Phe-Arg-MCA by urinary kallikrein is apparently inhibited with larger amounts of urine. Thus, the sample volume should not be larger than 20 μl. If urine shows a high kallikrein activity, such as, urine from Bartter's syndrome, the sample volume should be reduced to less than 20 μl. The sensitivity of the fluorogenic substrate method for the assay of urinary kallikrein is comparable with the radioimmunoassay method using plasma kininogen (73).

5.2. Brinase and brinase inhibitors

Brinase is a purified protease from Aspergillus oryzae and is being investigated as a potential thrombolytic agent.

It splits the substrate S 2160 and this property can be used to assess its level as well as the level of brinase inhibitors in plasma.

The following set up has been used (74, 75).

	Standard	Test
Tris/Imidazole buffer (pH 8.2, 50 mM, 0.1 M NaCl)	0.6 ml	0.55 ml
Brinase (0.1 Casein units/ml)	0.4 ml	0.4 ml
Plasma dilution in buffer 1:5		0.05 ml
Incubation for 5 min at 25°C after which		
Incubation mixture	0.25 ml	
Substrate solution 1 mM	0.25 ml	
Buffer	2.00 ml	

ΔA is continuously registered at 405 nm at 25°C.

Coefficient of variation 5%.

Because of the residual activity of the $\alpha_2 M$ inhibitor-brinase complex the results obtained with this method need not automatically be the same as those obtained with higher molecular weight substrates.

5.3. Bacterial endotoxins

The principle of the method is that bacterial endotoxin activates a clotting enzyme in the hemocyte lysate from the horseshoe crab (Tachypleus or limulus variety). The amidase activity of this enzyme can be measured with a chromogenic substrate.

Chromogenic substrates with the COOH-terminal sequence Gly-Arg-pNA are usually acceptable as substrates. The not commercially available substrates with the N-terminal sequences Boc-Val-leu, Boc-leu, Boc-Val-Ser-, and Boc-Ser (OBz)- are readily split. Of the commercially available ones, Chromozym UK is readily susceptible to the action of both the amidase activities arising from Tachpleus and limulus haemotcyte lysates.

No standardised method for the determination of bacterial endotoxin with chromogenic substrates has as yet been described (76, 77).

Fluorogenic substrate method for assay of bacterial endotoxins (78, 79)
(Contributed by S. Iwanaga, H. Kato, T. Morita, T. Sugo, Y. Ohno, M. Ohki, K. Takada, S. Sakakibara)

Principle: An endotoxin activated hemocyte lysate from the horseshoe crabs (*Tachypleus tridentatus and Limulus polyphemus*) hydrolyzes specifically Boc-Leu-Gly-Arg-MCA and this amidase activity is due to (an) endotoxin-sensitive clotting enzyme(s) contained in the lysate. The amidase activity increases by increasing the concentration of bacterial endotoxins added to the lysate (78). Therefore, the measurement of the endotoxin-induced amidase activity made it possible to determine the concentration of the endotoxin.

Reagents:

Limulus hemocyte lysate — A commercial preparation of hemocyte lysate from *Tachypleus tridentatus* (Japanese horseshoe crab), named Pregel® (Seikagaku Kogyo Co., Ltd., Tokyo), is used. One ampoule is dissolved in $270\,\mu l$ of Triz-HCl buffer, pH 8.0, (see below) before use, and the ampoule is placed in an ice bath.

Endotoxin: A commercial preparation of bacterial endotoxins, *E. coli* 0111: B4 (Difco Laboratories, Co.), is used as a standard endotoxin. One ampoule containing $1.0\,\mu g$ of endotoxin is dissolved in a pyrogen-free saline.

Buffer: 0.4 M Tris-HCl, pH 8.0, containing $0.04\,MgCl_2$ is prepared using a pyrogen-free distilled water from Otsuka Pharmaceutical Co., Tokyo.

Table IV.3.   Concentrations of some plasma proteins

	Molecular weight	Approximate conc.
Factor XII	80 000	450 nmol/l
Factor XII$_a$	80 000	
Factor XII$_b$	28 000	
Factor XI	170 000 (dimer)	30 nmol/l
Factor IX	70 000	70 nmol/l
Factor IX$_a$	45 000	
Factor VIII	2 000 000	
	(250 000 subun)	~ 50 nmol/l*
Factor VII	45 500	10 nmol/l
Factor VII$_a$	45 500	
Factor X	55 000	180 nmol/l
Factor X$_a$	45 000	
Factor V	300 000	25 nmol/l
Factor V$_a$	250 000	
Factor II	66 000	1 500 nmol/l
Factor II$_a$	36 600	
Factor XIII	350 000	
Factor XIII*	160 000	
Factor XIII$_a$	160 000	
Fibrinogen	360 000	10 000 nmol/l
Prekallikrein	100 000	1 100 nmol/l
Kallikrein	100 000	
Plasminogen	92 000	1 400 nmol/l
Plasmin	85 000	
Streptokinase	53 000	
Glandular kallikrein	25–35 000	
High molecular weight kallikrein	200 000	350 nmol/l
Low molecular weight kallikrein	60 000	2 000 nmol/l
Antithrombin III	65 000	2 000 nmol/l
α_2-antiplasmin	65 000	900 nmol/l
α_2-macroglobulin	750 000	3 500 nmol/l
α_1-antitrypsin	52 000	25 000 nmol/l
α_1-antichymotrypsin	65 000	7 000 nmol/l
inter-α-trypsin inhibitor	160 000	3 000 nmol/l
C^1-inhibitor	150 000	2 200 nmol/l

*three different concentrations were used (0.1, 0.05 and 0.01 mol/l).

Substrate: Boc-Leu-Gly-Arg-MCA is dissolved in pyrogen-free distilled water, to give a final concentration of 2.0 mM (1.6 mg/ml) and stored in a frozen state ($-20°$C).

Stopper: 12.5% acetic acid.

Procedure: The reaction mixture containing 50 μl of the substrate and 100 μl of endotoxin with different concentrations or unknown sample is preincubated at 37°C for 3 min. Then, 50 μl of Pregel® is added and the mixture incubated further for 15 min. After incubation, 100 μl of 12.5% acetic acid is added to terminate the reaction and the AMC released is measured.

Comments: The amidase activity determined fluorometrically increases by increasing concentration of endotoxin added to the hemocyte lysate, and a linear relationship between the toxin concentration and the activity is observed in the range of 5×10^{-6} to 5×10^{-2} μg of endotoxin. This method is at least fifty times more sensitive than the so called 'Limulus test' and is very reproducible. However, the method is not directly applicable for the assay of endotoxin in circulating blood, as the amidase activity is strongly inhibited by antithrombin III and α_2-plasmin inhibitor (80). Thus, some pretreatment with heat (56°C, 10 min) or chloroform is required before the assay on plasma samples (79).

References

1. Workman EF, Uhteg LC, Kingdon HS, Lundblad RL: In: Chemistry and Biology of Thrombin. Lundblad RL, Fenton JW, Mann KG (eds). Ann Arbor Science Publishers Inc., Ann Arbor, 1977, pp. 23–42
2. Gaffney PJ, Miller-Anderson M, Kirkwood TBL: Haemostasis 7:109–112 (1978)
3. Fenton JW, Landis BH, Walz DA, Finlayson JS: In: Chemistry and Biology of Thrombin. Lundblad RL, Fenton JW, Mann KG (eds). Ann Arbor Science Publishers Inc., Ann Arbor, 1977, pp. 43–70
4. Kirchhof BRJ, Vermeer C, Hemker HC: Thromb Res 13:219–232 (1978)
5. Jilek F, Lill H, Munz E: J Clin Chem 19:717 (1981) (meeting abstr.)
6. Bergström K, Egberg N: Thromb Res 12:531–547 (1978)
7. Bergström K, Blombäck M: Thrombos Res 4:719–729 (1974)
8. Axelsson G, Korsan-Bergtsen K, Waldenström J: Thromb Haemost 36:517–524 (1976)
9. Orthner CL, Morris S, Kosov DP: Thromb Res 23:533–539 (1981)
10. Abildgaard U, Lie M, Ødegard OR: Scand J Clin Lab Invest 36:109–112 (1976)
11. Abildgaard U, Lie M, Ødegard OR: Thromb Res 11:549–553 (1977)
12. Bergström K, Lahnborg G: Thromb Res 6:223–233 (1975)
13. Blombäck M, Blombäck B, Olsson P, Svendsen L: Thromb Res 5:621–632 (1974)
14. Mitchell GA, Hudson PM, Huseby RM, Pochron SP, Gargiulo RJ: Thromb Res 12:219–225 (1978)
15. Ødegard OR: Thromb Res 7:351–360 (1975)
16. Ødegard OR, Lie M, Abildgaard U: Thromb Res 6:287–294 (1975)
17. Ødegard OR, Rosenlund B, Ewik E: Haemost 7:202–209 (1978)
18. Vinazzer H: Haemost 4:101–109 (1975)
19. Rosing J, Tans G, Govers-Riemslag JWP, Zwaal RFA, Hemker HC: J Biol Chem 255:274–283 (1980)
20. Bevers EM, Comfurius P, van Rijn JLML, Hemker HC, Zwaal RFA: Eur J Biochem 122:429–436 (1982)
21. Morita T, Jackson CM: Thromb Haemostas 42:55 (1979)
22. Jesty J, Nemerson Y: J Biol Chem 249:509–515 (1974)
23. Lindhout MJ, Kop-Klaasen BHM, Hemker HC: Biochim Biophys Acta 533:327–341 (1978)
24. Vinazzer H, Heimburger N: Thromb Res 12:503–510 (1978)
25. Dieijen G van, Tans G, Rijn J van, Zwaal RFA, Rosing J: Biochemistry 20:7097–7101 (1981)
26. Aurell L, Friberger G, Karlsson G, Claeson G: Thromb Res 11:595–609 (1977)
27. van Wijk EM, Kahlé LH, Ten Cate JW: Clin Chem 26:885–890 (1980)
28. van Wijk EM, Kahlé LH, Ten Cate JW: Thromb Res 22: 681–686 (1981)

122

29. Ødegard OR, Lie M, Abildgaard U: Haemostasis 5:265–275 (1976)
30. Mattler LE, Bang NU: Thrombs Haemost 38:776–792 (1977)
31. Abildgaard U: In: Chromogenic Peptide Substrates. Chemistry and Clinical Usage. Scully MF, Kakkar VV (eds). Churchill Livingstone, London, 1979, pp. 171–179
32. Teien AN, Lie M: Thromb Res 10:399–410 (1977)
33. Holm HA, Abildgaard U, Laerum F, Wolland T: In: Synthetic Substrates in Clinical Blood Coagulation Assays. Lijnen HR, Collen D, Verstraete M (eds). Martinus Nijhoff Publishers, The Hague, 1980, pp. 63–67
34. Putten JJ van, Ruit M van de, Beunis M, Hemker HC: Clin Chem Acta 122: 261–270 (1982)
35. Bolton AE, Lundlam CA, Pepper DS, Moore S, Cash JP: Thromb Res 8:51–58 (1976)
36. Levine SP, Krentz LS: Thromb Res 11:673–686 (1977)
37. Andersen P, Godal HC: Haemostasis 6:339–346 (1977)
38. Gjesdal K: In: Chromogenic Peptide Substrates. Chemistry and Clinical Usage. Scully MF, Kakkar VV (eds). Churchil Livingstone, London, 1979, pp. 219–225
39. Vinazzer H: Haemost 6:283–293 (1977)
40. Vinazzer H: Haemost 7:352–358 (1976)
41. van Dieijen G, Tans G, Rosing J, Hemker HC: J Biol Chem 256:3433–3442 (1981)
42. Nemerson Y, Zur M, Bach R, Gentry RD: In: The Regulation of Coagulation. Mann KG, Taylor FB (eds). Elsevier North-Holland, New York, 1980, pp. 193–203
43. Seghatchian MJ, Miller-Andersson M: Med Lab Sci 35:347–354 (1978)
44. Tans G, Janssen-Claessen T, van Dieijen G, Hemker HC, Rosing J: accepted for publication in Thromb Haemostas
45. Dieijen-Visser MP van, Wersch P van, Brombacher P, Rosing J, Hemker HC, Dieijen G van: Haemostasis 12:241–255 (1982)
46. Østerund B, Rapaport SI: Proc Natl Acad Sci 12:5260–5264 (1974)
47. Fujikawa K, Legaz ME, Davie EW: Biochem 11:4882–4891 (1972)
48. Sandberg H, Andersson LO: Thromb Res 14:113–124 (1979)
49. Seligsohn U, Østerund R, Rapaport SI: Blood 52:978–988 (1978)
50. Poller L, Thomson JM, Bodzenta A, Easton AC, Latallo ZS, Chmielewska J: Br J Haematol 49:69–75 (1981)
51. Hemker HC, Muller AD, Gonggrijp R: J Molec Med 1:127–134 (1976)
52. Morrisson-Silverberg SA, Jesty J: J Biol Chem 256:1625–1630 (1981)
53. Wohl RC, Arzadon L, Summaria L, Robbins KC: J Biol Chem 252:1141–1147 (1977)
54. Wohl RC, Summaria L, Robbins KC: J Biol Chem 255:2005–2013 (1980)
55. Robbins KC, Wohl RC, Summaria L: In: Progress in Chemical Fibrinolysis. Vol. IV. Davidson JF, Cepelak V, Samaria MM, Desnoyens PC (eds). Churchill Livingstone, Edinburgh, 1979, pp. 330–338
56. Wohl RC, Summaria L, Arzadon L, Robbins KC: J Biol Chem 253:1402–1407 (1978)
57. Griffin JH: In: Haemostasis and Thrombosis. Bloom AL, Thomas DP (eds). Churchill Livingstone, London, 1981, pp. 84–97
58. Claeson G, Friberger P, Knös H, Eriksson E: Haemostasis 7:76–78 (1978)
59. Egberg N, Bergström K: Haemostasis 7:85–91 (1978)
60. Heber H, Geiger R, Heimburger N: Hoppe Seyler's Z Physiol Chem 359:659–669 (1978)
61. Stormorken H, Baklund A, Gallimore M, Rilaund S: Haemostasis 7:69–75 (1978)
62. Vinazzer H: Thromb Res 14:155–166 (1979)
63. Soulier JP, Gorin D: In: Advances in Biosciences. Haberland GL, Hamburg U (eds). Pergamon Press, Oxford, 1979, pp. 271

64. Kluft C: J Lab Clin Med 91:83—95 (1978)
65. Ogston D, Ogston CM, Ratnoff OD, Forbes CD: J Clin Invest 48:1786—1793 (1969)
66. Oh-ishi S, Katori M: Thromb Res 14:551—559 (1979)
67. Oh-ishi S, Webster ME: Biochem Pharmacol 24:591—598 (1975)
68. Sugo T, Ikari N, Kato H, Iwanaga S, Fuji S: Seikagaku (in Japanese) 51:589—595 (1979)
69. Fujikawa K, Kurachi K, Davie EW: Biochemistry 16:4182—4188 (1977)
70. Kato H, Maruyama I, Ohno Y, Sugo T, Iwanaga S: Seikagaku (in Japanese) 51:589—594 (1979)
71. Koide I, Kato H, Davie EW: Biochemistry 16:2279—2286 (1977)
72. Kato H, Adachi N, Iwanaga S, Abe K, Takada K, Kimura T, Sakakibara S: J Biochem 87:1127—1132 (1980)
73. Carretero OA, Oza NB, Piwonska T, Ocholik AG: Biochem Pharmacol 25:2265—2270 (1976)
74. Amundsen S: 10th International Congress on Thromb and Haemost. Vienna, Abstract p. 54, 1973
75. Nijman D, Duckert F: Thromb Diath Haemorrh. 33:221—225 (1975)
76. Nakamura S, Morita T, Iwanaga S, Niwa M, Takahasi T: J Biochem 81:1567—1569 (1977)
77. Iwanaga S, Morita T, Harada T, Nakamura S, Niwa M, Takada K, Kimura T, Sakakibara S: Haemost 7:183—188 (1978)
78. Harada T, Morita T, Iwanaga S: J Med Enz (in Japanese) 3:43—60 (1978)
79. Harada T, Ohki M, Niwa M, Iwanaga S: Thromb Baemost 42:109 (1979)
80. Harada T, Morita T, Iwanage S, Nakamura S, Niwa M: In: Biomedical applications of the Horseshoe Crab (Limulidal). Cohen E (ed). Alan R. Liss. Inc. New York, 1979, pp. 209—220

Bibliography on synthetic substrates (as available Fall 1982)

As an addendum we decided to present a list of the literature on substrates as available to us in the fall of 1982. The references are given in alphabetical order. To enable the reader to find quickly those articles he is interested in, each reference is provided with a code referring to the type of assay described and the substrate(s) used in it. The code consists of the letter(s) A (for assay) and/or S (for substrate), each followed by one or more ciphers; the ciphers following the letter A indicate the type of assay described and those following the letter S indicate the substrate(s) used. The translation of the code is to be found in the tables given below.

Table 1.   Relation between the assay code and the type of determination described

Assay code	Type of determination
A: 1.1	Thrombin
A: 1.2	Prothrombin
A: 1.3	Antithrombin III, heparin cofactor, heparin, antiheparins
A: 1.4	Prothrombinase, platelet factor 3
A: 1.5	Factor V
A: 2.1	Factor X_a
A: 2.2	Factor X
A: 2.3	Antithrombin III, heparin cofactor, heparin, antiheparins
A: 2.4	Factor X activating complex, platelet factor 3
A: 2.5	Factor IX, IX_a
A: 2.6	Factor VIII
A: 3.1	Plasmin
A: 3.2	Plasminogen
A: 3.3	Antiplasmin
A: 3.4	Plasminogen activators
A: 4.1	Plasma prekallikrein, plasma kallikrein, kallikrein inhibitors
A: 4.2	Factor XII, XII_a
A: 4.3	Factor XI, XI_a
A: 5.1	Glandular kallikrein, inhibitors of glandular kallikrein
A: 5.2	Brinase, Brinase inhibitors
A: 5.3	Bacterial endotoxins, Horseshoe crab clotting enzyme
A: 6	Other proteases
A: 7	General contemplation, kinetic study, review
A: 8	Chromogenic analogon of an overall clotting test
A: 9	Classification impossible for technical reasons

Examples: The code A: 2.2, S: 1. Means that in the article coded this way a determination of factor X using the chromogenic substrate S 2222 is described.

The code A: 7 means that the article does not give a description of a specific test, but has a more general character (general contemplation, kinetic study, review etc.).

Table 2. Relation between the substrate code and the substrate used

Substrate code	Substrate used
S: 1	S 2222
S: 2	S 2337
S: 3	S 2444
S: 4	Chromozym UK
S: 5	S 2266
S: 6	Chromozym PK
S: 7	S 2302
S: 8	S 2238
S: 9	Chromozym TH
S: 10	S 2288
S: 11	S 2160
S: 12	S 2251
S: 13	Chromozym PL
S: 14	S 2586
S: 15	S 2484
S: 16	Fluorogenic substrates
S: 17	Small ester substrates
S: 18	Thioester substrates
S: 19	Other chromogenic substrates, encountered rarely in the literature
S: 20	Substrates for electrochemical determinations
S: 21	Compounds giving an amplification of colour yield after the splitting of chromogenic substrates
S: 22	Luminogenic substrates

Bibliography on synthetic substrates (as available Fall 1982)
(Contributed by M.C.E. van Dam-Mieras)

Aasen AO, Frolich W, Saugstad OD, Amundsen E: Eur Surg Res 10:50–62, 1978.
Plasma kallikrein activity and prekallikrein levels during endotoxin shock in dogs.
A: 4.1, S: 6.
Aasen AO, Gallimore MJ, Ohlsson K, Amundsen E: Haemostasis 7:164–169, 1978.
Alterations of plasmin activity, plasminogen levels and activity of antiplasmins during endotoxin shock in dogs.
A: 3.1, 3.3, S: 12.
Aasen AO, Gallimore MJ, Lilleaasen P, Lyngaas K, Larsbraten M, Amundsen E: Eur Surg Res 11:145–153, 1980.
Changes in antiplasmin and plasmin activities during extreme hemodilution and open heart surgery in dogs.
A: 3.1, 3.3, S: 12.

Aasen AO, Larsbraaten M: *In* JF Davidson, RM Rowan, PC Samama, PC Desnoyers (eds). Progress in Chemical Fibrinolysiş and Thrombolysis Vol. 3. Raven Press, New York, 1978, pp 323–326.
'Immediate' and 'time-depending' antiplasmin activity in endotoxin shock in dogs.
A: 3.3, S: 12.

Abildgaard U: *In* MF Scully, VV Kakkar (eds). Chromogenic Peptide Substrates: Chemistry and Clinical Usage. Churchill Livingstone, London, 1979, pp 171–179.
Antithrombin assays using chromogenic substrates.
A: 1.3, 2.3, S: 1, 8, 11.

Abildgaard U: *In* MF Scully, VV Kakkar (eds). Chromogenic Peptide Substrates: Chemistry and Clinical Usage. Churchill Livingstone, London, 1979, pp 229–234.
Chromogenic substrates in the control of anticoagulant therapy.
A: 2.3, S: 1.

Abildgaard U, Lie M, Ødegard OR: Scand J Clin Lab Invest 36:109–112, 1976.
A simple amidolytic method for the determination of functionally active antithrombin III.
A: 1.3, S: 11.

Abildgaard U, Lie M, Ødegard OR: Thromb Res 11:549–553, 1977.
Antithrombin (heparin-cofactor) assay with 'new' chromogenic substrates (S 2238 and chromozym TH).
A: 1.3, S: 8, 9.

Abildgaard U, Lie M, Teien A, Ødegard OR: Thromb Diath Haemorrh 34:345, 1975. Thromb Haem Vth Congr, Paris, Abstract.
Coagulation inhibitors studied with chromogenic substrate.
A: 1.3, S: 11.

Adams RW, Elmore DT: Biochem J 124:66P–67P, 1972.
The kinetics of hydrolysis of synthetic substrates by bovine factor XA.
A: 7, S: 17.

Aguinebeitia MJ, Iriard JA: Thrombos Haemost (Stuttgart) 45:188, 1981.
Automation of a kinetic factor X assay.
A: 2.2, S: 2.

Aiach M, Kher A, Mardignian J: Thrombos Haemostas 42:381, 1979 (Meeting abstract).
Hog and beef mucosal heparin – in vitro study using different assay procedures.
A: 2.3.

Aiach M, Schreiber N, Nussas C, Michaud A, Léon M, Lederc M: Thromb Res 21: 317–320, 1981.
An automated amidolytic assay for testing factor X activity.
A: 2.2, S: 1.

Aiyappa PA: Thrombos Haemostas 46:350, 1981 (Meeting abstract).
Involvement of factor VII in intrinsic coagulation pathway: synthetic substrate assay for coagulation factor activities in plasma.
A: 8, S: 19.

Aiyappa PA: Ann NY Acad 370:812–821, 1981.
Chromogenic substrate spectrophotometric assays for the measurement of clotting function.
A: 8, S: 19.

Amundsen E: 10th International Congress on Thrombosis and Haemostasis, Vienna, 1973, p 54 (Meeting abstract).
A: 9.

Amundsen E, Aasen AO, Gallimore MJ, Larsbraaten M, Lyngaas K: *In* MF Scully, VV Kakkar (eds). Chromogenic peptide substrates: Chemistry and Clinical Usage. Churchill Livingstone, Edinburgh, 1979, pp 72–82.
The plasma-kallikrein-kinin system in endotoxin shock in dogs.
A: 4.1.

128

Amundsen E, Putter J, Friberger P, Knös M, Larsbraten M, Claeson G: *In* S Fujii, H Moriya, T Suzuki (eds). KININS-II: Biochemistry, Pathophysiology and Clinical Aspects. Plenum Publishing Corporation, 1979, pp 83−95.
Methods for the determination of glandular kallikreins by means of a chromogenic tripeptide substrate.
A: 5.1, S: 5.
Amundsen E, Svendsen L: *In* I Witt (ed). New methods for the analysis of coagulation using chromogenic substrates. de Gruyter, Berlin, 1977, pp 211−219.
A new assay for plasma kallikrein activity utilizing a synthetic chromogenic substrate.
A: 4.1, S: 6.
Amundsen E, Svendsen L, Vefling A: IVth Int Congr Thrombosis and Haemostasis, Vienna, 1973 (Meeting abstract 22).
A sensitive photometric method for determination of plasma inhibition towards plasmin and Brinase.
A: 3.3.
Amundsen E, Svendsen L, Vennerød AM, Laake K: *In* Pisano and Austen. Chemistry and Biology of the Kallikrein-Kinin System in Health and Disease. Fogarty Int Center Publ no 27 US Printing Office, Washington, 1976, pp 215−220.
Determination of plasma kallikrein with a new chromogenic tripeptide derivative.
A: 4.1, S: 6.
Andersen P: Haemostasis 9:303−309, 1980.
The antiheparin effect of α_1-acid glycoprotein, evaluated by the activated partial thromboplastin time and by a factor X_a assay for heparin.
A: 2.3, S: 1.
Andreasen T: Haemostasis 9:65−70, 1980.
Automated two-stage assay for determination of antithrombin III with a centrifugal analyzer.
A: 1.3, S: 8.
Arocha-Piñango CL, Pepper DS: Thrombos Haemostas 46:710−713, 1981 (Meeting abstract).
Studies of a fibrinolytic enzyme from the larvae of Lonomia achelons (Cramer) using chromogenic peptide substrates.
A: 7, S: 1, 3, 7, 12.
Aurell L, Claeson G, Karlsson G, Friberger P: *In* Proc of the 14th European peptide symposium Weipon Belgium Ed de l'Université de Bruxelles, 1976, pp 191−195.
Chromogenic substrates based on the primary structure of prothrombin − especially intended for the determination of factor X_a activity.
A: 7.
Aurell L, Friberger P, Karlsson G, Claeson G: Thromb Res 11:595−609, 1977.
A new sensitive and highly specific chromogenic peptide substrate for factor X_a.
A: 2.1, 2.2, S: 1.
Aurell L, Gustavsson S, Friberger P: Thrombos Haemostas 46:342, 1981 (Meeting abstract).
Chromogenic substrates and activated forms of FXII: comparison between α- and β-forms and selectivity with regard to plasma kallikrein and FXI_a.
A: 4.2, S: 1, 7.
Aurell L, Olaussen A, Claeson G: Thromb Diath Haemorrh 34:591, 1975 (Meeting abstract).
Determination of factor X_a activity by means of chromogenic substrates based on the primary structure of prothrombin.
A: 2.1, S: 1.
Aurell L, Simonsson R, Arielly S, Karlsson G, Friberger P, Claeson G: Haemostasis 7:92−94, 1978.
New chromogenic peptide substrates for factor X_a.
A: 2.1, S: 1.

Avvisati G, Ten Cate JW, van Wijk EM, Kąhlé LH, Mariani G: Brit J Haem 45:343–352, 1980.
Evaluation of a new chromogenic assay for factor VII and its application in patients on oral anticoagulant treatment.
A: 2.4, S:1.

Axelsson G, Korsan-Bengtsen K, Waldenström J: Thrombos Haemostas (Stuttgart) 36:517–524, 1976.
Prothrombin determination by means of a chromogenic peptide substrate.
A: 1.2, S: 1, 2.

Baba S, Takizawa N, Nakaniski K, Igaraski M: Blood and Vessel (Japan) 12:490–492, 1981.
Determination of α_2-plasmin inhibitor with chromogenic peptide substrate.
A: 3.3, S: 13.

Baele G: In HR Lijnen, D Collen, M Verstraete (eds). Synthetic Substrates in Clinical Blood Coagulation Assays. Martinus Nijhoff, Publishers, The Hague, 1980, pp 37–42.
Spectrophotometric determination of factor X with S 2222 in anticoagulated and cirrhotic patients.
A: 2.2, S: 1.

Bajaj SP, Rapaport SI, Brown SF: J Biol Chem 256:253–259, 1981.
Isolation and characterization of human factor VII. Activation of factor VII by factor X_a.
A: 2.4, S: 1.

Bang NU, Mattler LE: In RL Lundblad, JWII Fenton, KG Mann (eds). Chemistry and Biology of Thrombin. Ann Arbor Science Publishers, Ann Arbor, 1977, pp 305–310.
Thrombin sensitivity and specificity of the the chromogenic peptide substrates.
A: 1.1, 2.1, S: 1, 8, 9, 11.

Bang NU, Mattler LE: Haemostasis 7:98–104, 1987.
Sensitivity and specificity of plasma serine protease chromogenic substrates.
A: 2.3, 3.2, 3.3, 4.1, S: 1, 6, 8, 11, 12.

Barlow GH, Marder VJ: Thromb Res 18:431–437, 1981.
Plasma urokinase levels measured by chromogenic assay after infusions of tissue culture or urinary source material.
A: 3.4, S: 3.

Barrowcliffe TW, Johnson EA, Eggleton CA, Kemball-Cook G, Thomas DP: Br J Haematol 41:573–583, 1979.
Anticoagulant activities of high and low molecular weight heparin fractions.
A: 2.3, S: 1.

Bartl K: Thromb Res 13:1141–1142, 1978.
Effect of heparinbinding to thrombin on thrombin activity measured with a chromogenic substrate.
A: 1.1, S: 9.

Bartl K, Lill H: Thromb Res 18:267–272, 1980.
A versatile assay method of antithrombin III using thrombin and Tos-Gly-Pro-Arg-pNA.
A: 1.3, S: 9.

Baughman DJ, Lytwyn A: Thrombos Haemostas 42:291, 1979 (Meeting abstract).
A novel chromogenic assay equivalent to the one stage prothrombin time (PT).
A: 8, S: 8.

Baughman DJ, Raritan NJ, Natelsòn EA, Triplett DA, Zimmerman TS: Thrombos Haemostas 42:291, 1979 (Meeting abstract).
Characteristics of amidolytic antithrombin III (AT) assay.
A: 1.3, S: 8.

130

Bergström K: LKB Application Note 211.
Determination of trypsin in duodenal fluid using a new chromogenic substrate and a reaction rate instrument.
A: 6.
Bergström K, Blombäck M: Thromb Res 4:719—729, 1974.
Determination of plasma prothrombin with a reaction rate analyzer using a synthetic substrate.
A: 1.2, S: 11.
Bergström K, Egberg N: Thromb Res 12:531—547, 1978.
Determination of vitamin K sensitive coagulation factors in plasma: studies on three methods using synthetic chromogenic substrates.
A: 1.2, 1.4, 2.2, S: 1, 8.
Bergström K, Lahnborg G: Thromb Res 6:223—233, 1976.
The effect of major surgery, low doses of heparin and thromboembolism on plasma antithrombin. Comparison of immediate thrombin inhibiting capacity and the antithrombin III content.
A: 1.3, S: 11.
Bertina RM, Loeliger EA: In HR Lijnen, D Collen, M Verstraete (eds). Synthetic Substrates in Clinical Blood Coagulation Assays. Martinus Nijhof Publishers, The Hague, 1980, pp 13—23.
The potential use of chromogenic assays in the routine monitoring of oral anti-coagulant therapy.
A: 1.2, 2.2, S: 1, 2, 8.
Bertina RM, Loeliger EA: Thrombos Haemostas 46:328, 1981 (Meeting abstract).
Definition and evaluation of a therapeutic range for the control of oral anti-coagulant treatment by chromogenic assays.
A: 1.2, 2.2.
Bertina RM, van der Marel-van Nieuwkoop W, Loeliger EA: Thrombos Haemostas 42:226, 1979 (Meeting abstract).
Spectrophotometric assays of prothrombin in plasmas of patients on oral anti-coagulants.
A: 1.2.
Bevers EM, Comfurius P, van Rijn JLML, Hemker HC, Zwaal RFA: Europ J Biochem 122:429—436, 1982.
Generation of platelet prothrombin converting activity and the exposure of phos-phatidylserine at the platelet outer surface.
A: 1.4, S: 8.
Bhargava AS, Heinick J, Schöbel Chr, Günzel P: Thrombos Haemostas 42:381, 1979 (Meeting abstract).
A comparison of anticoagulation activity of a potent heparin preparation in different test.
A: 1.1, 2.1, S: 1, 8.
Bhargava AS, Schöbel C, Günzel P: Arzneimittelforsch 31:79—82, 1981.
Characterization of a new potent heparin. 6th communication: The comparison of the anticoagulant effect of the sodium and calcium salts of a new potent heparin after s.c. injection in beagle dogs.
A: 2.3, S: 1.
Bick RL, Arbegast NR: Thrombos Haemostas 46:21, 1981 (Meeting abstract).
A comparison of chromogenic, fluorogenic and fibrinogen substrate assays for the determination of plasma heparin.
A: 1.3, S: 8, 16.
Bick RL, McClain BJ: Thrombos Haemostas 46:364, 1981 (Meeting abstract).
A clinical comparison of chromogenic, fluorometric and natural (fibrinogen) substrate assays for determination of antithrombin-III.
A: 7.

Bigbee WL, Jensen RH: Biochim Biophys Acta 540:285–294, 1978.
Characterization of plasminogen activator in human cervical cells.
A: 3.4, S: 16.

Binder BR, Spragg J: Blut 40:38, 1980 (Meeting abstract).
Plasminogenaktivierung durch Urokinase (UK) und durch den vasculären Plasmino-
gen Aktivator (VPA). Einfluss von Fibrinogen und Thrombin.
A: 3.4, S: 12.

Bishop RC, Hudson PM, Mitchell GA, Pochron SP: Ann NY Acad 370:720–730,
1981.
Use of fluorogenic substrates for the assay of anti-thrombin-III and heparin.
A: 1.3, S: 16.

Blaskó GY: Prostaglandins 18:3–9, 1980.
Effects of PGI_2 on the inactivation of thrombin, factor X_a, and plasmin by
antithrombin-III and heparin.
A: 1.3, 2.3, 3.3, S: 1, 9, 12.

Blombäck M, Blombäck B, Olsson P, Svendsen L: Thromb Res 5:621–632, 1974.
The assay of antithrombin using a synthetic chromogenic substrate for thrombin.
A: 1.3, S: 11.

Blombäck B, Hessel B, Hogg D, Claeson G: In RL Lundblad, JW Fenton, KG Mann
(eds). Chemistry and Biology of Thrombin. Ann Arbor Science Publisher Inc
Ann Arbor, Mich., 1977, pp 275–290.
Substrate specificity of thrombin on proteins and synthetic substrates.
A: 7.

Bodzenta A, Thomson JM, Latallo ZS: Thrombos Haemostas 46:363, 1981 (Meeting
abstract).
An assessment of an amidolytic assay for factor VII in the laboratory control
of oral anticoagulants.
A: 7.

Bönner G, Marin-Grez M: J Clin Chem Clin Biochem 19:165–168, 1981.
Measurement of kallikrein activity in urine of rats and man using a chromogenic
tripeptide substrate. Validation of the amidolytic assay by means of bradykinin
radioimmunoassay.
A: 5.1, S: 5.

Bokarev IN, Butorov VN, Loginov LE: Ter Arkh 53:118–124, 1981.
Primenenie khromogennykh substratov dlia diagnostiki narusheni'i svertyvaniia
krovi i fibrinoliza. (Use of chromogenic substrates for the diagnosis of blood
coagulation and fibrinolytic disorders).
A: 9.

Borsodi A, Machovich R: Act Physl H 52:277, 1978 (Meeting abstract).
Inactivation of alpha-thrombins and beta-thrombins by plasma inhibitors .3.
amidolytic and esterolytic activities of alpha-thrombins and beta-thrombins.
A: 1.1, 1.3, S: 11, 17.

Borsodi A, Machovich R: Biochim Biophys Acta 566:385–389, 1979.
Inhibition of esterase and amidase activities of α and β-thrombin in the presence
of antithrombin III and heparin.
A: 1.1, 1.3, S: 11.

Bounameaux H, Duckert F: In I Witt (ed). New Methods for the Analysis of Coagulation using Chromogenic Substrates. de Gruyter, Berlin, 1977, pp 57–59.
A: 7, S: 9, 11.

Bounameaux H, Marbet GA, Airenne H, Grossmann E, Stanojevic B, Eichlisberger R,
Lämmle B, Duckert F: Thrombos Haemostas 42:380, 1979 (Meeting abstract).
Control of heparin treatment with three different methods. Behaviour of anti-
thrombin III.
A: 7, S: 1.

Branchini BR, Hermes JH, Salituro FG, Post NP, Claeson G: Anal Biochem 111:87–96, 1981.
Sensitive enzyme assays based on the production of chemiluminescent leaving groups.
A: 7, S: 22.

Branchini BR, Salituro FG, Hermes JD, Post NJ: Bioch Biophys Res Comm 97:334–339, 1980.
Highly sensitive assays for proteinases using immobilized luminogenic substrates.
A: 7, S: 22.

Brandt JT, Triplett DA, Schaeffer J: Thrombos Haemostas 46:341, 1981 (Meeting abstract).
The effect of different activators and thromboplastins on a chromogenic APTT.
A: 8.

Briel RC: Blut 40:80, 1980. (Meeting abstract).
Gerinnungsphysiologische Untersuchungen mit chromogenen Substraten bei low-dose Heparin und Heparin/Dihydroergotamin-Prophylaxe.
A: 1.3, 2.3, 3.3, S: 1, 8, 12.

Briel RC, Wagner U, Weselek R, Kunz S: Thrombos Haemostas 42:380, 1979 (Meeting abstract).
Heparin levels using the chromogenic substrate S 2222 during low dose heparin and low dose heparin-dihydroergotamin-prophylaxis after gynecological surgery.
A: 2.3, S: 1.

Brown JE, Baugh RF, Hougie C: Thromb Res 17:267–272, 1980.
The inhibition of the intrinsic generation of activated factor X by heparin and hirudin.
A: 2.4, S: 1.

Byrne R, Link RP, Castellino FJ: J Biol Chem 255:5336–5341, 1980.
A kinetic evaluation of activated bovine blood coagulation of factor IX toward synthetic substrates.
A: 7, S: 17.

Carmignota F, Schivo P, Zotti S, Ceriotti G: Arch Sci Med (Torino) 137:467–470, 1981.
L'AT III in patologia epatica. Confronto tra la determinazione immunologica e quella con substrato cromogeno. (At III in liver diseases. Comparison between immunological determination and that with chromogenic substrate).
A: 1.3, S: 9.

Casis E, Aguinebeitia MJ, Iriarte JA: Thrombos Haemostas 45:188, 1981 (short note).
Automation of a kinetic factor-X assay.
A: 2.2, S: 2.

Castillo MJ, Nakajima K, Zimmerman M, Powers JC: Anal Biochem 99:53–64, 1979.
Sensitive substrates for human leukocyte and procine pancreatic elastase: a study of the merits of various chromophoric and fluorogenic leaving groups in assays of serine proteases.
A: 7.

Cate JW ten: In HR Lijnen, D Collen, M Verstraete (eds). Synthetic Substrates in Clinical Blood Coagulation Assays. Martinus Nijhoff Publishers, The Hague, 1980, pp 45–50.
An automated chromogenic antithrombin III method: Clinical experience.
A: 1.3, S: 8.

Cate JW ten, Lamping RJ, Kahlé LH: Paramedica 10:29–33, 1980.
Klinische relevantie van bepalingen met chromogene substraten.
A: 7.

Chester A, Crawford GP: Clin Exp PH 8:361, 1981 (Meeting abstract).
Amidolytic measurement of normal prothrombin using a fraction of tiger snake-venom as activator.
A: 1.2, S: 9.

Chmielewska J, Teisseyre E, Raczka E, Mussoni L, Donati MB, Latallo ZS: *In* JF Davidson (ed). Progress in Chemical Fibrinolysis and Thrombolysis Vol. IV. Churchill Livingstone, London, 1979, pp 167—170.
Evaluation of various components of the fibrinolytic system in man and laboratory animals with the use of chromogenic substrates.
A: 3.2, 3.3, 3.4, S: 12.

Choo IHF, Didisheim P, Doerge ML, Johnson ML, Bach ML, Melchert LM, Johnson NJ, Taylor WF: Thromb Res 25:115—123, 1982.
Evaluation of a heparin assay-method using a fluorogenic synthetic peptide substrate for thrombin.
A: 1.3, S: 16.

Ciavarella N, Coccheri S, Gensini GF, Hassan HJ, Mannucci PM, Manotti C, Margstakler E, Mariani G. Orlando M, Palareti G, Petronelli M, Pogliani E, Ponari O, Prisco D, Recalcati P, Rosse E, Salvitti C, Tripodi A: Thromb Res 19:493—502, 1981.
Multicenter evaluation of a new chromogenic factor X assay in plasma of patients on oral anticoagulants.
A: 2.2, S: 2.

Christensen U: Thrombos Haemostas 43:169—174, 1980.
Requirements for valid assays of clotting enzymes using chromogenic substrates.
A: 7.

Christensen U, Ipsen HH: Biochem Biophys Acta 569:177—183, 1979.
Steady-state kinetics of plasmin- and trypsin-catalysed hydrolysis of a number of tripeptide-p-nitroanilides.
A: 7.

Christensen U, Ipsen HH: Thrombos Haemostas 42:453, 1979 (Meeting abstract).
The steady state kinetics of plasmin and trypsin catalyzed hydrolysis of a number of tripeptideanilides.
A: 7.

Christensen U, Sottrup-Jensen L, Magnusson S, Peterson TE, Clemmensen I: Biochim Biophys Acta 567:472—481, 1979.
Enzymic properties of the neo-plasmin-Val-442 (miniplasmin).
A: 7, S: 11, 12, 17.

Claeson G, Aurell L: Ann NY Acad Sci 370:798—811, 1981.
Small synthetic peptides with affinity for proteases in coagulation and fibrinolysis an overview.
A: 7.

Claeson G, Aurell L, Friberger P, Gustavsson S, Karlsson G: Haemostasis 7:62—68, 1978.
Designing of peptide substrates. Different approaches exemplified by new chromogenic substrates for kallikreins and urokinase.
A: 7.

Claeson G, Aurell L, Karlsson G, Friberger P: *In* I Witt (ed). New Methods for the Analysis of Coagulation using Chromogenic Substrates. de Gruyter, Berlin, 1977, pp 37—54.
Substrate structure and activity relationship.
A: 7.

Claeson G, Aurell L, Karlsson G, Friberger P: *In* CJF Davidson, RM Rowan, MM Samama, PC Desnoyers (eds). Chemical Fibrinolysis and Thrombolysis. Vol. 3. Raven Press, New York, 1978, pp 299—304.
Substrate structure and activity relationship.
A: 7.

134

Claeson G, Aurell L, Karlsson G, Gustavsson S, Friberger P, Arielly S, Simonsson R: *In* MF Scully, VV Kakkar (eds). Chromogenic Peptide Substrates: Chemistry and Clinical Usage. Churchill Livingstone, London, 1979, pp 20—30.
Design of chromogenic peptide substrates.
A: 7.
Claeson G, Ekenstam B, Aurell L, Arwin H, Lundström I: Haemostasis 7:135—136, 1978.
New electric method to determine enzymatic activity. Determination of anti-thrombin in whole blood.
A: 7.
Claeson G, Friberger P, Knös H, Eriksson E: Haemostasis 7:76—78, 1978.
Methods for determination of prekallikrein in plasma, glandular kallikrein and urokinase.
A: 3.4, 4.1, 5.1, S: 5, 7, 19.
Clark SE, Scully MF, Webb P, Kakkar VV: Thrombos Haemostas 42:110, 1979 (Meeting abstract).
Measurement of endotoxin levels in plasma using Limulus amoebocyte lysate and chromogenic substrate, S 2222.
A: 5.3, S: 1.
Clavin SA, Bobbitt JL, Shuman RT, Smithwich EL Jr: Anal Biochem 80:355—365, 1977.
Use of peptidyl-4-methyoxy-2-naphtylamides to assay plasmin.
A: 3.1, S: 16.
Coen D, Bini A, Balconi G, Delaini F, Mussoni L, Donati MB: Thrombos Haemostas 46:64, 1981 (Meeting abstract).
Plasminogen activator (PA) activity in metastatic cells: an amidolytic approach.
A: 3.4, S: 12.
Coleman PL, Green GDJ: Meth Enzym 80 (PC): 408—424, 1981.
A coupled photometric assay for plasminogen activator.
A: 3.4, S: 18.
Collen D, Edy J, Wiman B: *In* MF Scully, VV Kakkar (eds). Chromogenic Peptide Substrates: Chemistry and Clinical Usage. Churchill Livingstone, London, 1979, pp 238—244.
Discrimination between antiplasmins: reaction mechanisms, biological role and assay of the fast acting plamin inhibitor in human plasma.
A: 3.3, S: 12.
Collen D, Lijnen HR, De Cock F, Durieux JP, Loffet A: Biochim Biophys Acta 615: 158—166, 1980.
Kinetic properties of tripeptide lysyl chloromethyl ketone and lysyl p-Nitroanilide derivatives towards tyrpsin-like serine proteinases.
A: 7.
Colucci M, Curatolo L, Donati MB, Semerano N: Thromb Res 18 (3—4): 589—595, 1980.
Cancer cell procoagulant activity: evaluation by an amidolytic assay.
A: 2.4, S: 1.
Conard J, Barbier P, Samama M: Thrombos Haemostas 42:1350—1352, 1979.
Automated amidolytic method for AT-III determination.
A: 1.3, S: 8.
Conard J, Gradelet A, Samama M: Ann Biol Clin 39:81—83, 1981.
Dosage du facteur Stuart a l'aide d'un substrat synthétique au cours des traitements anticoagulants oraux. Resultats prelininaires.
A: 2.2, S: 2.
Cullman W, Adler K, Müller PN: Thrombos Haemostas 42:34, 1979 (Meeting abstract).
Factor XII assay in plasma with the chromogenic substrate 'chromozym PK'.
A: 4.2, S: 6.

Czapek EE, Kwaan HC, Szczecinski M: J Lab Clin Med 95:783–790, 1980.
The effect of a sulfated polysaccharide on antithrombin III.
A: 1.3, 2.3, 3.3, S: 1, 8, 12.

Daraio de Peuriot M, Nigretto JM, Jozefowicz M: Thromb Res 20:299–306, 1980.
Electrochemical activity determination of trypsinlike enzymes .3. Application
to the assay of antithrombin-III in aqueous-solutions, human-plasma and whole
blood.
A:1.3, S: 20.
Daraio de Peuriot M, Nigretto JM, Jozefowicz M: Thromb Res 22:303–308, 1981.
Electrochemical activity determination of trypsin-like enzymes .4. Coupled electro-
chemical and spectrophotometric assay of thrombin using the same H-D-Phe-Pip-
Arg-4 MEO Beta-Naphtyl-Amide, 2 HCl (S 2421) substrate.
A: 1.1, S: 16.
Daraio de Peuriot M, Nigretto JM, Jozefowicz M: Thrombos Res 19:647–654, 1980.
Electrochemical activity determination of trypsin-like enzymes. II.-thrombin.
A: 1.1, S: 20.
Dettori AG, Civardi E, Magni R, Fenik D, Ponari O: Thrombos Haemostas 42:20,
1979 (Meeting abstract).
Automated kinetic assay for antithrombin III with a chromogenic substrate.
A: 1.3, S: 9.
Diaz-Cremades JM, Vicente JM, Borrell M, Felez J, Gimferrer E, Pujal N, Domingo A,
Rutlant ML: Sangre 23:347–357, 1978.
Determinación de un nuevo inhibidor de la fibrinólisis usando substratos chromo-
génicos: la antiplasmina rápida.
A: 3.3, S: 12.
Dick W, Cullman W, Muller N: Z. Anal. Chem. 311:452–453, 1982 (Meeting abstract).
Evaluation of a new amidolytic factor-X assay — its automation and its relation
to standard procedures.
A: 7.
Dick W, Cullman W, Muller N, Adler K: J Clin Chem 19:357–361, 1981.
Factor XII assay with the chromogenic substrate chromozym PK.
A: 4.2, S: 6.
Dieijen G, Tans G, Rijn J van, Zwaal RFA, Rosing J: Biochemistry 20:7096–7101,
1981.
Simple and rapid method to determine the binding of blood clotting factor X to
phospholipid vesicles.
A: 7, S: 1.
Dieijen G van, Tans G, Rosing J, Hemker HC: J Biol Chem 256:3433–3442, 1981.
The role of phospholipid and factor VIII alpha in the activation of bovine factor
X.
A: 7, S: 1.
Dieijen-Visser MP van, Wersch J van, Brombacher P, Rosing J, Hemker HC, Dieijen G
van: Haemostasis 12:241–255, 1982.
Use of chromogenic peptide substrates in the determination of clotting factors,
II, VII, IX and X in normal plasma of patients with oral anticoagulants.
A: 1.2, 2.2, 2.4, 2.5, S: 2, 9.
Dombrose FA, Bode AP, Sandberg H, Lentz BR, Jones ME, Crumpler DC: Thrombos
Haemostas 46:341, 1981 (Meeting abstract).
Platelet factor V-like coagulant activity and catalytic phospholipid-like surface
activity in clotting and chromogenic assays.
A: 1.4, S: 8.
Dooijewaard G, Kluft C: Thrombos Haemostas 46:63, 1981 (Meeting abstract).
Generation of factor XII-dependent plasminogen activator activity in human
plasma measured with a fluorogenic substrate.
A: 3.4, S: 16.

136

Dooijewaard G, Kluft C: Thrombos Haemostas 46:390, 1981 (Meeting abstract).
The estimation of α-antiplasmin by means of synthetic substrates; kinetic analysis and optimization of the method.
A: 3.3.
Downing MR, Bloom JW, Mann KG: Biochemistry 17:2649–2653, 1978.
Comparison of the inhibition of thrombin by three plasma protease inhibitors.
A: 1.3, S: 11.
Droulle C, Lafaurie M, Remy MG, Florent B, Potron G: Thrombos Haemostas 46:363, 1981 (Meeting abstract).
Problems raised by the measurement of coagulation factors on chromogen substrates by automatic methods.
A: 7.
Duckert F: Aktuelle Diagnostik. Boehringer Mannheim 1976.
Die Anwendung chromogener Substrate in der Gerinnungsanalytik.
A: 7.
Duckert F: Med Lab (Stuttgart) 32:25–32, 1979.
Die chromogenen Substrate. Ihre diagnostische Anwendungen in der Gerinnung und Fibrinolyze.
A: 7.
Duckert F, Marbert GA: Annales Biologie Clinique Med Hyg 35:911, 1977.
Le contrôle du traitement aux anticoagulants oraux. La zone therapeutique.
A: 7.
Duckert F, Witt I, Svendsen L: In Chromogenic Substrates in Coagulation Analysis. Boehringer Mannheim, 1977.
A: 7.
Duncan A, Bowie EJW, Owen CA Jr: Thrombos Haemostas 46:313, 1981 (Meeting abstract).
Automated coagulation factor assays using a thrombin specific chromogenic substrate.
A: 8.
Dunikoski LK, Myrmel KH, Derzack MT: Clin Chem 25:1076, 1979 (Meeting abstract).
Automated chromogenic antithrombin-III assay with a centrifugal analyzer.
A: 1.3, S: 8.

Ebert Ch, Beller FK: Blut 40:60, 1980 (Meeting abstract).
Zur Biochemie des menstrualblutes.
A: 9, S: 1, 7, 8, 11, 12.
Edlefson DS, Aiyappa PA: Thrombos Haemostas 46:344, 1981 (Meeting abstract).
Evaluation of contact activation of the intrinsic coagulation system in evacuated tubes: chromogenic substrate assay equivalent to the non-activated partial thromboplastin time.
A: 8.
Edy J, De Cock F, Collen D: Thrombosis Research 8:513–518, 1976.
Inhibition of plasmin by normal and antiplasmin-depleted human plasma.
A: 3.3, S: 12.
Edy J, Collen D, Verstraete M: Abstr 3rd Int Conf on Synthetic Fibrinolytic Thrombolytic Agents, Glasgow, Sept 1979.
Quantitation of the plasma protease inhibitor antiplasmin with the chromogenic substrate S 2251.
A: 3.3, S: 12.
Edy J, Collen D, Verstraete M: In JF Davidson, RM Rowan, MM Samama, PC Desnoyers (eds). Progress in Chemical Fibrinolysis and Thrombolysis 3. Raven Press, New York, 1978, pp 315–322.

Quantitation of the plasma protease inhibitor antiplasmin with the chromogenic substrate S 2251.
A: 3.3, S: 12.
Egberg N, Bergström K: *In* MF Scully, VV Kakkar (eds). Chromogenic Peptide Substrates: Chemistry and Clinical Usage. Churchill Livingstone, London, 1979, pp 61–67.
Synthetic chromogenic substrates in the assay for plasma prekallikrein and coagulation factors II and X.
A: 1.2, 1.4, 2.2, 4.1, S: 1, 7, 8.
Egberg N, Bergström K: Haemostasis 7:85–91, 1978.
Studies on assays for plasma prekallikrein and for the monitoring of coumarol therapy.
A: 1.2, 1.4, 2.2, 4.1, S: 1, 7, 8.
Egberg N, Heedman PA: Thromb Res 25:437–440, 1982.
Simplified performance of amidolytic factor X assay. S 2337 and S 2222.
A: 2.2, S: 1, 2.
Egberg N, Johnsson H: Thrombos Haemostas 46:297, 1981 (Meeting abstract).
Experience of control of the initiation of coumarol therapy with an amidolytic assay of factor X.
A: 2.2, S: 1.
Egbring R, Menche B, Fuchs F, Jacobi J, Heimburger N, Havemann K: Thrombos Haemostas 42:225, 1979 (Meeting abstract).
Antithrombin III determination by an amidolytic method before and after ATIII substitution.
A: 9.
Elödi P, Pozgay M, Bajusz S, Simonsson R: Thrombos Haemostas 42:19, 1979 (Meeting abstract).
A method for designing chromogenic substrates for thrombin.
A: 7.
Engelberg H, Lee S: Thrombos Haemostas 46:375, 1981 (Meeting abstract).
Endogenous heparin activity in normal human plasma.
A: 2.3.
Eriksson E, Friberger P: Thrombos Haemostas 42:460, 1979 (Meeting abstract).
A chromogenic antithrombin assay with a recently introduced test kit optimization and titration of reagents.
A: 1.3, S: 11.
Eriksson E, Rosén S, Knös M, Friberger P: Thrombos Haemostas 46:315, 1981 (Meeting abstract).
Chromogenic substrate methods for the determination of $FVIII_c$, endotoxin and plasminogen activator.
A: 2.4, 3.4, 5.3, S: 1, 10, 12, 19.
Erskine JG, Walker ID, Davidson JF: J Clin Pathol 33:445–448, 1980.
Maintenance control of oral anticoagulant therapy by a chromogenic substrate assay for factor X.
A: 2.2, S: 2.
Erskine JG, Walker ID, Davidson JF: Clin Lab H 4:179–186, 1982.
Maintenance control of oral anticoagulant therapy by an automated chromogenic substrate assay of factor X.
A: 2.2, S: 2.
Estelles A, Aznar J, Gilabert J, Parrilla JJ: Pediatr Res 14:1180–1185, 1981.
Dysfunctional plasminogen in full-term newborn.
A: 3.2, S: 12.

Famodu AA, Ingram GIC: Clin Lab H 4:27–39, 1982.
Oral anticoagulant control with a chromogenic substrate: calibration, precision and cost.
A: 7.

Famodu AA, Ingram GIC, Darby SC: Thrombos Haemostas 42:292, 1979 (Meeting abstract).
Anticoagulant control with chromogenic measurements of factors X and VII.
A: 2.2, S: 1.

Fareed J, Kindel G, Messmore HL, Balis JU: In GL Haberland, U Hamberg (eds). Current Concepts in Kinin Research. Pergamon Press, Oxford, 1979, pp 237–247.
A: 9.

Fareed J, Messmore HL, Balis JU: In MF Scully, VV Kakkar (eds). Chromogenic Peptide Substrates: Chemistry and Clinical Usage. Churchill Livingston, London, 1979, pp 183–191.
Current status of methodologies for antithrombin III and heparin with the advent of peptide chromogenic substrates.
A: 1.3, 2.3, S: 1, 8.

Fareed J, Messmore HL, Bermes EW: Clin Chem 26:1380–1391, 1981.
New perspectives in coagulation testing.
A: 1.3, 2.3, 3.2, 3.3, 7, S: 1, 2, 8, 9, 12.

Fareed J, Messmore HL, Gallagher J, Orfei P, Parvez Z, Fenton J: Thrombos Haemostas 42:206, 1979 (Meeting abstract).
Inhibition of thrombin by H-D-Pro-Phe-Arg-OH (S 2430), H-D-Pro-Phe-Arg-NH$_2$ (S 2443) H-D-Phe-Phe-Arg-NH$_2$ (S 2448) and their derivatives.
A: 7.

Fareed J, Messmore HL, Kindel G, Balis JU: Ann NY Acad Sci 370:765–784, 1981.
Inhibition of serine proteases by low molecular weight peptides and their derivatives.
A: 7.

Fareed J, Messmore HL, Orfei R, Gallagher J, Parvez Z, Bermes EW: Clin Chem 25:1076, 1979 (Meeting abstract).
Comparative studies of the chromogenic substrate methodologies for the measurement of heparin-cofactor (Antithrombin-III).
A: 1.3, S: 8, 9, 11.

Fareed J, Messmore HL, Parvez Z, Orfei P, Gallagher J, Fenton JW: Thrombos Haemostas 42:400, 1979 (Meeting abstract).
Serine protease inhibition by low molecular weight peptides and their derivatives.
A: 7, S: 19.

Fareed J, Messmore HL, Walenga JM, Kniffin J, Bermes EW, Mariani G: Clin Chem 27:1107, 1981 (Meeting abstract).
Status of amidololytic methods for the laboratory monitoring anti-thrombotic, and procoagulant therapy.
A: 7.

Fareed J, Walenga J, Kelly J, Bernes EW, Messmore HL: Clin Chem 28:1586, 1982 (Meeting abstract).
Newer synthetic chromogenic substrates in hemostatic testing – comparative evaluation of antithrombin III, plasminogen, prekallikrein, alpha-2-antiplasmin, factor X and heparin methods.
A: 7.

Fareed J, Walenga JM, Kniffen JM, Messmore HL: Am J Med T 46:654, 1981.
Evaluation of some newer amidolytic assays for coagulation testing.
A: 8.

Farmer DA, Hageman JH: J Biol Chem 250:7366–7371, 1975.
Use of N-benzoyl-L-tyrosine thiobenzyl ester as a protease substrate.
A: 6, S: 17.

Fässler H, Duckert F, Marbet GA: Haemostasis 7:158–163, 1978.
Assay with chromogenic substrates of in vivo activated proteases.
A: 7.

Fässler H, Walter M, Marbet G, Duckert F: *In* I Witt (ed). New Methods for the Analysis of Coagulation using Chromogenic Substrates. de Gruyter, Berlin, 1977, pp 249–250.
The quantitative determination of urokinase with chromozym UK.
A: 3.4, S: 4.

Feinman RD, Chang TL, Wilson SM, Li EHH: *In* RL Lundblad, JW Fenton II, KG Mann (eds). The Chemistry and Biology of Thrombin. Ann Arbor Science publ inc. Ann Arbor, Michigan, 1977, p 217–232.
Application of rapid kinetic methods to thrombin reactions with substrates and antithrombin III.
A: 7.

Ferry JP: Feuillets de biologie XIX:19–24, 1978.
Dosage du facteur II plasmatique sur substrat chromogénique.
A: 1.2, S: 8.

Fiessinger JN, Aiach M, Nursas C, Capron L: Thrombos Haemostas 46:297, 1981 (Meeting abstract).
Kinetic study of factor X (FX): potential value for the initiation of oral anti-coagulant treatment.
A: 9.

Firkin BG, Goh A, Broadway M, Howard M: Thrombos Haemostas 42:20, 1979 (Meeting abstract).
The use of the chromogenic substrate S 2238 in the study of thrombin generation.
A: 1.4, S: 8.

Fisher CA, Schmaier AH, Addonizi VP, Colman RW: Blood 59:963–970, 1982.
Assay of prekallikrein in human plasma – comparison of amidolytic esterolytic coagulation and immunochemical assays.
A: 4.1, S: 7, 17.

Francis JL: J Clin Path 32:651–654, 1979.
New chromogenic assay for the specific determination of prothrombin.
A: 1.2, S: 9.

Fredin HO, Tengborn L: Thrombos Haemostas 46:373, 1981 (Meeting abstract).
Changes in biologically and immunochemically measured antithrombin III (AT III) in total hip replacement with special regard to type of thromboembolic prophylaxis.
A: 1.3, S: 8.

Friberger P, Axelson G, Korsan-Bengsten K: Thromb Diath Haemorrh 34:321, 1975 (Meeting abstract).
Determination of plasminogen by means of a chromogenic peptide substrate.
A: 3.2, S: 11.

Friberger P, Claeson G, Knös M, Aurell L, Arielly S, Simonsson R: *In* JF Davidson (ed). Progress in Chemical Fibrinolysis and Thrombolysis, vol. 4. Churchill Livingstone, Edinburgh, 1979, pp 149–153.
Activity of plasminogen activators on tripeptide chromogenic substrates.
A: 7.

Friberger P, Egberg N, Holmer E, Hellgren M, Blombäck M: Thromb Res 25:433–436, 1982.
Antithrombin assay – the use of human or bovine thrombin and the observation of a 'second' heparin cofactor.
A: 1.3, S: 8.

Friberger P, Eriksson E, Gustavsson S, Claeson G: *In* S Fujii, H Moriya, T Suzuki (eds). KININS-II: Biochemistry, Pathophysiology and Clinical Aspects. Plenum Publishing Corporation, New York, 1979, pp 67–82.

Determination of prekallikrein in plasma by means of a chromogenic tripeptide substrate for plasma kallikrein.
A: 4.1, S: 6, 7.

Friberger P, Knös M: *In* MF Scully, VV Kakkar (eds). Chromogenic Peptide Substrates. Chemistry and Clinical Usage. Churchill Livingstone, London, 1979, pp 128–139.
Plasminogen determination in human plasma.
A: 3.2, S: 12.

Friberger P, Knös M: *In* HR Lijnen, D Collen, M Verstraete (eds). Synthetic Substrates in Clinical Blood Coagulation Assays. Martinus Nijhoff Publishers, The Hague, 1980, pp 73–92.
Functional assays of the components of the fibrinolytic system using a plasmin sensitive substrate – a review.
A: 3.1, 3.2, 3.3, 3.4, S: 12.

Friberger P, Knös M, Gustavsson S, Aurell L, Claeson G: Thrombos Haemostas 38:22, 1977 (Meeting abstract).
Methods for the determination of plasmin, antiplasmin and plasminogen by means of the substrate S 2251.
A: 3.1, 3.2, 3.3, S: 12.

Friberger P, Knös M, Gustavson S, Aurell L, Claeson G: Haemostasis 7:138–145, 1978.
Methods for determination of plasmin, antiplasmin and plasminogen by means of substrate S 2251.
A: 3.1, 3.2, 3.3, S: 12.

Friberger P, Knös M, Gustavsson S, Aurell L, Claeson G: *In* MF Scully, VV Kakkar (eds). Chromogenic Peptide Substrates: Chemistry and Clinical Usage. Churchill Livingstone, London, 1979, pp 121–127.
A new specific substrate for the determination of plasmin activity.
A: 7, S: 12.

Friberger P, Lenne C: Thrombos Haemostas 42:54, 1979 (Meeting abstract).
A chromogenic factor X assay with new standardized reagents.
A: 2.2, S: 2.

Friedman RB, Kwaan HC, Srczecinski M: Thrombos Haemostas 38:20, 1977 (Meeting abstract).
Amplification of color yield obtained using a chromogenic substrate for determining plasminogen activator.
A: 3.4, S: 21.

Friedman RB, Kwaan HC, Srczecinski M: Thromb Res 12:37–46, 1977.
Improved sensitivity of chromogenic substrate assays for urokinase and plasmin.
A: 3.1, 3.4, S: 21.

Frigola A, Angeloni S, Cerqueti AR: J Clin Path 32:21–25, 1979.
Determination of anti-thrombin activity by an amidolytic and a clotting procedure.
A: 1.3, S: 9.

Fujikawa K, Kurachi K, Davie EW: Biochemistry 16:4182–4188, 1977.
Characterization of bovine Factor XII$_a$ (activated Hageman factor).
A: 4.2, S: 11.

Fuijwara K, Tsuru D: J Biochem 83:1145–1149, 1978.
New chromogenic and fluorogenic substrates for pyrorridonyl peptidase.
A: 6.

Fukuda C, Iijima K, Nakamura K: Rinsho Byori 29:179–182, 1981.
Clinical evaluations of antithrombin III and alpha-2-plasmin inhibitor assay method with chromogenic substrates (S 2238, S 2251 (author's transl)).
A: 1.3, 3.3, S: 8, 12.

Gaffney PJ: *In* MF Scully, VV Kakkar (eds). Chromogenic Peptide Substrates. Chemistry and Clinical Usage. Churchill Livingstone, London, 1979, pp 42—49.
A critical evaluation of chromogenic substrates in standardisation.
A: 7.

Gaffney PJ, Lord K, Brasher M, Kirkwood TBL: Thromb Res 10:549—556, 1977.
Problems in the assay of thrombin using synthetic peptides as substrates.
A: 1.1, S: 9, 11.

Gaffney PJ, Miller-Andersson M, Kirkwood TBL: Haemostasis 7:109—112, 1978.
Unreliability of chromogenic substrates for assay of the clotting activity of thrombin.
A: 1.1, S: 8, 9.

Gallimore MJ: Throm Res 17:289—291, 1980.
Inhibition of the amidolytic activity of urokinase by human plasma.
A: 3.4, S: 6.

Gallimore MJ, Amundsen E, Aasen AO, Larsbraaten M, Lyngaas K, Svendsen K: Thromb Res 14:51—60, 1979.
Studies on plasma antiplasmin activity using a new plasmin specific chromogenic tripeptide substrate.
A: 3.3, S: 13.

Gallimore MJ, Amundsen E, Larsbraaten M, Lyngaas K, Fareid E: Thrombos Haemostas 42:263, 1979 (Meeting abstract).
Chromogenic peptide substrate assays for plasma inhibitors of plasma kallikrein: identification of the major inhibitors.
A: 4.1.

Gallimore MJ, Fareid E: *In* MF Scully, VV Kakkar (eds). Chromogenic Peptide Substrates. Chemistry and Clinical Usage. Churchill Livingstone, London, 1979, pp 248—261.
Studies on human plasma inhibitors of plasmin, plasma kallikrein, trypsin, thrombin and urokinase using chromogenic substrate assays.
A: 1.3, 3.3, 4.1, 5.1, 6, S: 4, 6, 9, 12.

Gallimore MJ, Fareid E, Stormorken H: Thromb Res 12:409—420, 1978.
The purification of a human plasma kallikrein with weak plasminogen activator activity.
A: 4.1, S: 6.

Gallimore MJ, Friberger P: Thrombos Haemostas 46:314, 1981 (Meeting abstract).
Simple chromogenic peptide substrate assays for determining components of the plasma kallikrein system.
A: 4.1.

Gallimore MJ, Friberger P: Thromb Res 25:293—298, 1982.
Simple chromogenic peptide substrate assays for determining prekallikrein, kallikrein inhibition and kallikrein 'like' activity in human plasma.
A: 4.1, S: 7.

Gallimore MJ, Larsbraaten M, Lyngaas K, Fareid E: *In* JF Davidson (ed). Progress in Chemical Fibrinolysis and Thrombolysis vol. IV. Churchill Livingstone, London, 1979, pp 159—163.
A chromogenic substrate assay for plasma inhibitors of urokinase and the partial purification of the major inhibitor.
A: 3.4, S: 4.

Galluzzo TS, Tsao CH: Thromb Res 25:237—244, 1982.
Evaluation of a thrombin-sensitive fluorogenic substrate for heparin concentration in plasma.
A: 1.3, S: 16.

Gandolfo GM, De Angelis A, Torresi MV: Haemostasis 9:15—19, 1980.
Determination of antithrombin III activities by different methods in diabetic patients.
A: 1.3, S: 9.

Gauvin G, Umlas J: Am J Clin P 78:271, 1982 (Meeting abstract).
Measurements of plasma heparin levels using a fluorometric assay.
A: 1.3, S: 16.

Gibelli A: Minerva Med 69:1241–1244, 1978.
Determination of antithrombin III (Chromogenic substrates) and FDP in women in treatment with oral estroprogestin agents.
A: 1.3, S: 9.

Girolami A, Patrassi G, Toffanin F, Saffin L: Am J Clin Pathol 74:83–87, 1980.
Chromogenic substrate (S 2238) prothrombin assay in prothrombin deficiencies and abnormalities. Lack of identity with clotting assays in congenital dysprothrombinemias.
A: 1.2, S: 8.

Girolami A, Saggin L, Boeri G: Am J Clin Pathol 73:400–402, 1980.
Factor X assays using chromogenic substrate S 2222.
A: 2.2, S: 1.

Gjesdal K: In MF Scully, VV Kakkar (eds). Chromogenic Peptide Substrates. Chemistry and Clinical Usage. Churchill Livingstone, London, 1979, pp 219–225.
Platelet factor 4 and antiheparin activity in plasma.
A: 1.3, 2.3, S: 1, 8.

Goldsmith GH Jr: J Lab Clin Med 96:222–231, 1980.
Contact activated fibrinolysis: role of surface concentration and high-molecular-weight kininogen.
A: 3.1, 4.1.

Goldsmith GH, Stern RC, Saito H, Ratnoff OD: J Lab Clin Med 89:131–134, 1977.
Normal plasma arginine esterase and the Hageman factor (factor XII)-prekallikrein-kininogen system in cystic fibrosis.
A: 3.1, 4.1, S: 19.

Goodnight SH Jr, Schaeffer JL, Sheth K: Am J Clin Pathol 73:639–647, 1980.
Measurement of antithrombin III in normal and pathologic states using chromogenic substrate S 2238. Comparison with immunoelectrophoretic and factor X_a inhibition assays.
A: 1.3, S: 8.

Gray AJ, Uhlmeyer KA, Fedor EJ: Clin Chem 25:1147, 1979 (Meeting abstract).
Quantichrom AT III-chromogenic substrate assay for antithrombin III.
A: 1.3.

Gray AJ, Uhlmeyer KA, Fedor EJ: Thrombos Haemostas 42:225, 1979 (Meeting abstract).
Quantichrom AT III: diagnostic kit for the quantification of total antithrombin III activity in plasma.
A: 1.3.

Green GDJ, Shaw E: Anal Biochem 93:223–226, 1979.
Thiobenzyl Benzyloxicarbonyl-L-Lysinate, substrate for a sensitive colorimetric assay for trypsin-like enzymes.
A: 6, S: 17.

Griffith MJ: Thromb Res 25:245–253, 1982.
Measurement of the heparin enhanced-antithrombin III/thrombin reaction rate in the presence of synthetic substrate.
A: 7, S: 9.

Griffith MJ, Kingdon HS, Lundblad RL: Thromb Res 17:83–90, 1980.
Hydrolysis of N-α-benzoyl-L-Phenylalanyl-L-Valyl-L-Arginine-p-nitroanilide by human alpha thrombin in the presence of heparin.
A: 1.1, S: 11.

Gustavsson S, Aurell L, Karlsson G, Friberger P: Thrombos Haemostas 38:22, 1977 (Meeting abstract).

Chromogenic peptide substrates for kallikreins and urokinase.
A: 7.
Gyzander E, Friberger P, Myrwold H, Noppa H, Ohlsson R, Teger-Nilsson AC, Wallmo L: *In* I Witt (ed). New Methods for the Analysis of Coagulation using Chromogenic Substrates. de Gruyter, Berlin, 1977, pp 229–245.
Antiplasmin determination by means of the plasmin specific substrate S-2251-Methodological studies and some clinical applications.
A: 3.3, S: 12.
Gyzander E, Teger-Nilsson AC: Thromb Res 19:165–175, 1980.
Activity of the α_2-macroglobulin-plasmin complex on the plasmin specific substrate H-D-Val-Leu-Lys-p-nitroanilide.
A: 3.3, S: 12.

Harada T, Morita T, Iwanaga S: J Med Enz 3:43–60, 1978. (Jap.).
A new assay method for bacterial endotoxins using horseshoe crab clotting enzyme.
A: 5.3.
Harada T, Morita T, Iwanaga S, Nakamura S, Niwa M: *In* E Cohen (ed). Biomedical Applications of the Horseshoe Crab (Limulidal). Alan R Liss. Inc, New York, 1979, pp 209–220.
A new chromogenic substrate for assay of bacterial endotoxins using Limulus hemocyte lysate.
A: 7.
Harada T, Ohki M, Niwa M, Iwanaga S: Thrombos Haemostas 42:109, 1979 (Meeting abstract).
A new fluorogenic substrate method for assay of bacterial endotoxins using Limulus hemocyte lysate.
A: 5.3, S: 16.
Harada-Suzuki T, Morita T, Iwanaga S, Nakamura S, Niwa M: J Biochem 92:793–800, 1982.
Further studies on the chromogenic substrate assay method for bacterial endotoxins using horseshoe crab. (*Tachypleus tridentatus*) hemocyte lysate.
A: 7.
Hársfalvi J, Chmielewska J, Latallo ZS, Muszbek L: Thrombos Haemostas 46:315, 1981 (Meeting abstract).
Measurement of platelet factor 3 availability by using chromogenic substrate.
A: 1.4, S: 8.
Harsfalvi J, Chmielewska J, Latallo ZS, Muszbek L: J Clin Chem Clin Biochem 19:693, 1981 (Meeting abstract).
Measurement of platelet factor 3 availability using chromogenic substrate.
A: 1.4, S: 8.
Hasegawa H, Oguma Y, Takei H, Seya T, Yamauchi M, Murakoshi T, Nagata H, Murao M: Jpn Heart J 21:367–380, 1980.
Assay of heparin in plasma using a chromogenic substrate and its clinical applications.
A: 2.3, S: 1.
Hayashi S, Yamada K: Thromb Res 22:573–578, 1981.
Assay of urokinase activity in plasma with a chromogenic substrate. (S 2444).
A: 3.4, S: 3.
Heber H, Geiger R, Heimburger N: Hoppe Seyler's Z Physiol Chem 359:659–669, 1978.
Human plasma kallikrein: purification, enzyme characterization and qualitative determination in plasma.
A: 4.1, S: 6.

144

Heber H, Karges HE, Gehlert R, Debus R, Heimburger N: Blut 40:69, 1980 (Meeting abstract).
Antithrombin III − Bestimmung aus Plasma am Beispiel des neuen Chromogenen Thrombin-Substrat H-D-Phe-Pro-Arg-Leu-pNA.
A: 1.3, S: 19.
Heck L, Rosenberg R, Remold H: Prep Biochem 9:359−377, 1980.
Purification and properties of Guniea pigs antithrombin III.
A: 1.1, 1.3, S: 11.
Herrmann RP, Bailey PE: Thrombos Haemostas 41:544−552, 1979.
Plasma thrombin assay using a chromogenic substrate in disseminated intravascular coagulation due to snake bite envenomation.
A: 1.1, S: 9.
Hesse R, Tritschler W, Castelfranchi G, Bablok W: Blut 42:227−234, 1981.
Antithrombin III: Referenzwerte mit einem chromogenen Substrat (Chromozym TH).
A: 1.3, S: 9.
Higgins DL, Shafer JA: Anal Biochem 83:408−415, 1977.
An immobilized naphtylamide substrate for proteinases with tryptic-like specificity.
A: 1.1, 6, 7, S: 16.
Hiyikata A, Okamoto S, Kikumoto R, Tamao Y: Thrombos Haemostas 42:1039−1045, 1980.
Kinetic studies on the selectivity of a synthetic thrombin-inhibitor using synthetic peptide substrates.
A: 7, S: 1, 11, 12, 19.
Hitomi Y, Kanda T, Niinobe M, Fujii S: Clin Chim A 119:157−164, 1982.
A sensitive colorimetric assay for thrombin, prothrombin and antithrombin-III in human plasma using a new synthetic substrate.
A: 1.1, 1.2, 1.3, S: 19.
Hitomi Y, Niinobe M, Fujii S: Clin Chim Acta 100:275−283, 1980.
A sensitive colorimetric assay for human urinary kallikrein.
A: 5.1, S: 19.
Hojima Y, Tankersley DL, Miller-Andersson M, Pierce JV, Pisano JJ: Thromb Res 18:417−430, 1981.
Enzymatic properties of human Hageman factor fragment with plasma prekallikrein and synthetic substrates.
A: 7.
Holm HA, Abildgaard U, Laerum F, Wolland T: In HR Lijnen, D Collen, M Verstraete (eds). Synthetic Substrates in Clinical Blood Coagulation Assays. Martinus Nijhoff Publishers, The Hague, 1980, pp 63−67.
Heparin concentration (S 2222) and effect of heparin treatment (bleeding complications, pulmonary embolism and clearing of the thrombus).
A: 7, S: 1.
Hughes DR, Faust RJ, Didisheim P, Tinker JH: Anesth Anal 61:189−190, 1982 (Meeting abstract).
Heparin monitoring during cardiopulmonary bypass in man − use of fluorogenic heparin assay to validate activated clotting time.
A: 1.3, S: 16.
Hurlet-Birk Jensen A, Maes E, Gillet C, Legrand-Monsieur A: Thrombos Haemostas 43:104−107, 1981.
Reliability of amidolytic assays for progressive antithrombin and heparin cofactor activities on capillary blood.
A: 7.
Huseby RM, Clavin SA, Smith RE, Hull RN, Smithwick EL Jr: Thromb Res 10:679−687, 1977.
Studies on tissue culture plasminogen activator. II. The detection and assay of

urokinase and plasminogen activator from LLC-PK Cultures (porcine) by the synthetic substrate N-alpha-Benzyloxycarbonyl-Glycyl-Glycyl-Arginyl-4-Methoxy-2-Napthylamide.
A: 3.4, S: 16.

Huseby RM, Smith RE: Seminars in thrombosis and hemostasis VI 173−314, 1980.
Synthetic oligopeptide substrates: Their diagnostic application in blood coagulation, fibrinolysis and other pathologic states.
A: 7.

Ito R, Statland BE: Clin Chem 27:586−593, 1981.
Centrifugal analysis for plasma kallikrein activity, with use of the chromogenic substrate S 2302.
A: 4.1, S: 7.

Iwanaga S, Kato H, Maruyama I, Adachi N, Ohno Y, Takada K, Kimura T, Sakakibara S: Thrombos Haemostas 42:49, 1979 (Meeting abstract).
Fluorogenic peptide substrates for proteases in blood coagulation kallikrein-kinin and fybrinolysis systems: substrate for plasmin and factor XI_a.
A: 7, S: 16.

Iwanaga S, Morita T, Harada T, Nakamura S, Niwa M, Takada K, Kimura T, Sakakibara S: Haemostasis 7:183−188, 1978.
Chromogenic substrates for horseshoe crab clotting enzyme. Its application for the assay of bacterial endotoxins.
A: 5.2, S: 1, 4, 19.

Iwanaga S, Morita T, Kato H, Harada T, Adachi N, Sugo T, Maruyama I, Takada K, Kimura T, Sakakibara S: In S Fujii, H Moriya, T Suzuki (eds). Kinins-II, Biochemistry, Pathophysiology and Clinical Aspects. Plenum Publ Corp, New York, 1979, pp 147−163.
Fluorogenic peptide substrates for proteases in blood coagulation, kallikrein-kinin, and fibrinolysis systems.
A: 7, S: 16.

Iwanaga S, Morita T, Kato H, Harada T, Adachi N, Sugo T, Maruyama I, Takada K, Kimura T, Sakakibara S: Adv Exp Med Biol 120A:147−163, 1980.
Fluorogenic peptide substrates for proteases in blood coagulation, Kallikrein-kinin and fibrinolysis systems.
A: 7, S: 16.

Jackson CM: Thrombos Heamostas 42:458−459, 1979 (Meeting abstract).
Synthetic peptide substrates − biochemical evaluation.
A: 7.

Jackson CM: Thrombos Haemostas 46:328, 1981 (Meeting abstract).
Prospects for chromogenic and fluorogenic substrate use in biochemistry and blood protease assay.
A: 7.

Jering H, Jilek F, Lill H, Roeschlau P: J Clin Chem Clin Biochem 19:717, 1981 (Meeting abstract).
A photometric assay for determination of α_2-antiplasmin.
A: 3.3, S: 13.

Jilek F, Lill H, Munz E: J Clin Chem Clin Biochem: 19:717, 1981 (Meeting abstract).
Experience with a versatile photometric assay for prothrombin in plasma.
A: 1.2, S: 9.

Jonker JJC, Riel LHM van, Paulssen MMP: Thrombos Haemostas 42:446, 1979 (Meeting abstract).
Comparison of a new automated amidolytic assay of thrombin generation with 'prothrombin time' and 'thrombotest'.
A: 8, S: 9.

Jürgens H, Voss H von, Göbel U: Klin Paediatr 192:330—335, 1981.
Die Bestimmung von Inhibitoren der Haemostase mit chormógenen Substraten.
A: 1.3, 2.3, 3.3, S: 1, 8, 12.

Kahlé LH, Jenkins CSP, Ali-Briggs E, ten Cate JW: Thromb Res 13:645— 653, 1978.
Antithrombin III. II. comparison of different substrates and thrombin preparation.
A: 1.3, S: 8, 9, 11.
Kahlé LH, Lamping RJ, ten Cate JW: Thrombos Haemostas 42:48, 1979 (Meeting abstract).
Evaluation of an automated amidolytic antiplasmin assay.
A: 3.3.
Kahlé LH, Lamping RJ, ten Cate JW: Paramedica 9:5—9, 1980.
Klinisch chemische aspecten van geautomatiseerde chromogene stollingsbepalingen.
A: 7.
Kahlé LH, Schipper HG, Jenkins CSP, ten Cate JW: Thromb Res 12:1003—1014, 1978.
Antithrombin III. I. Evaluation of an automated antithrombin III method.
A: 1.3, S: 9.
Kanaoka Y, Takahashi T, Nakayama H: Chem Pharm Bull 25:362—363, 1977.
A new fluorogenic substrate for aminopeptidase.
A: 6, S: 16.
Kapke GF, Feld RD, Witte DL, Johnson GF: Clin Chem 28:1521—1524, 1982.
Single-stage automated-assay for heparin. (technical note)
A: 1.3, S: 16.
Kapke GF, Johnson GF, Witte DL, Feld RD: Clin Chem 27:1107, 1981, (Meeting abstract).
Automated fluorometric heparin assay on the multistat-III.
A: 1.3, S: 16.
Karges HE, Heber H, Heimburger N: Blut 40:37, 1980 (Meeting abstract).
Neue chromogene Substrate zur Bestimmung von Gerinnungsenzymen und anderen Serinproteasen.
A: 7.
Kato H, Adachi N, Iwanaga S, Abe K, Takada K, Kimura T, Sakakibara S: J Biochem (Tokyo) 87:1127—1132, 1980.
A new fluorogenic substrate method for the estimation of kallikrein in urine.
A: 5.1, S: 16.
Kato H, Adachi N, Ohno Y, Iwanaga S, Takada K, Sakakibara S: J Biochem (Tokyo) 88:183—190, 1981.
New fluorogenic peptide substrates for plasmin.
A: 3.1, S: 16.
Kato H, Fujimahi M, Fukutake K: Thrombos Haemostas 42:105, 1979 (Meeting abstract).
Studies on nature of so-called antiplasmin measured by chromogenic substrate S 2251 and its automatic determination with ABA 100.
A: 3.3, S: 12.
Kato H, Maruyama I, Ohno Y, Sugo T, Iwanaga S: Seikagaku (in Japanese) 51:589, 1979.
Role of HMW kinogen in Hageman factor-mediated activation of factor XI.
A: 4.3, S: 16.
Kato H, Nagatsu T, Kimura T, Sakakibara S: Seikgaku (In Japanese) 49:990, 1979.
A: 6. S: 16.
Kato H, Sugo T, Ikari N, Hashimoto N, Mazuyama I, Hau YN, Iwanaga S, Fujii S: In S Fujii, H Moriya, T Suzuki (eds). Kinins-II, Synthetic Proteases and Cellular Functions. Plenum Publ Corp, New York, 1979, pp 19—37.

Role of bovine high-molecular-weight (HMW) kininogen in contact mediated activation of bovine factor XII.
A: 9, S: 16.

Kiesewetter H, Eschweiler H, Pütz H, Frömel M, Angelkort B, Schmid-Schönbein H: Blut 40:92, 1980 (Meeting abstract).
Ein abstimmbarer Farbstofflaser zur mikrophotometrischen Erfassung der Aktivierung von Gerinnungsenzymen mit synthetischer Substraten.
A: 1.1, 2.1.

Kindness G, Long WF, Williamson FB: Br J Pharmacol 68:645—649, 1980.
Evidence for antithrombin III involvement in the anticoagulant activity of cellulose sulphate.
A: 7, S: 1, 11.

Kirchhof BRJ, Muller AD, Vermeer C, Hemker HC: Haemostasis 8:1—7, 1979.
Control of anticoagulant therapy with a chromogenic substrate.
A: 1.2, S: 9.

Kirchhof BRJ, Vermeer C, Hemker HC: Thromb Res 13:219—232, 1978.
The determination of prothrombin using synthetic chromogenic substrates; choice of a suitable activator.
A: 1.2, S: 8, 9.

Klauser RJ, Blümel G: Blut 40:53, 1980 (Meeting abstract).
Probleme der Kallikreinbestimmung in Urin.
A: 5.1, S: 5.

Klausner YS, Rigbi M, Ticho T, de Jong PJ, Negiusky EJ, Rinott Y: Biochem J 169:157—167, 1978.
The interaction of alpha-N-(p-toluenesulphonyl)-p-guanidino-L-phenylalanine methyl ester with thrombin and trypsin.
A: 7.

Klessen C, Sturzebecher J, Markward F: Thromb Res 25:501—505, 1982.
Determination of factor XII in plasma using the kallikrein substrate chromozym-PK (technical note).
A: 4.2, S: 6.

Kluft C: Thesis. Dutch Efficiency Bureau. Pijnacker, 1978, p 104.
Preactivators and activators in human plasma.
A: 7.

Kluft C, Trumpi-Kalshoven MM, Jie AFH: In MF Scully, VV Kakkar (eds). Chromogenic Peptide Substrates: Chemistry and Clinical Usage. Churchill Livingston, London, 1979, pp 84—92.
Crucial conditions for the determination of prekallikrein levels in plasma with chromogenic substrates.
A: 4.1, S: 6, 7.

Knos M, Friberger P: In JF Davidson (ed). Progress in Chemical Fibrinolysis and Thrombolysis vol. IV. Churchill Livingstone, London, 1979, pp 154—158.
Methods for plasminogen determination in human plasma and for streptokinase standardisation.
A: 3.2, 3.4, S: 12.

Köhler M, Hellstern P, Wenzel E: Blut 42:131, 1981 (Meeting abstract).
Verleichende Untersuchungen der Fibrin(ogen)olyze mit amidolytischen, immunologischen Verfahren und einem neuen lasterturbidimetrischen Prinzip.
A: 3.1, 3.4, S: 3, 13.

Kohn S, Sakurama S, Morioka T, Ito Y, Yasukouchi T, Nakagawa S: Thrombos Haemostas 42:1261—1275, 1980.
The interaction between heparin and plasmin on amidolysis.
A: 3.1, S: 17.

Korsan-Bengtsen K, Axelsson G: Thromb Diath Haemorrh 34:939, 1975 (Meeting abstract).

Prothrombin determination by means of a chromogenic peptide substrate.
A: 1.2, S: 11.
Korsan-Bengtsen K, Axelsson G, Waldenström J: *In* I Witt (ed) New Methods for the Analysis of Coagulation using Chromogenic Substrates. de Gruyter , Berlin, 1977, pp 145–154.
Determination of plasma prothrombin with the chromogenic peptide substrate H-D-Phe-Pip-Arg-pNA (S 2238).
A: 1.2, S: 8.
Korsan-Bengtsen K, Christenson B, Andersson I, Johnsen M: Thrombos Haemostas 42:56, 1979, (Meeting abstract).
Platelet factor 3 availability during platelet clumping – studied with a method based on a chromogenic peptide substrate.
A: 1.4, S: 8.
Kosow DD: Biochemistry 14:4459–4465, 1975.
Kinetic mechanism of the activation of human plasminogen by streptokinase.
A: 3.4, S: 17.
Kosow DP, Furie BC, Forastieri H: Thromb Res 4:219–227, 1974.
Activation of factor X: Kinetic properties of the reaction.
A: 2.2, S: 17.
Kwaan HC, Friedman RB, Szczecinski M: Thromb Res 13:5–13, 1978.
Amplification of color yield of chromogenic substrates using p-Dimethylamino-cinnamaldehyde.
A: 3.4, S: 21.

Lämmle B, Bounameaux H, Marbet GA, Eichlisberger R, Duckert F: Thrombos Haemostas 44:150–153, 1981.
Monitoring of oral anticoagulation by an amidolytic factor X assay. A long-term study in 42 patients.
A: 2.2, S: 1.
Lämmle B, Duckert F: Thrombos Haemostas 43:112–117, 1981.
Different assessment of plasmin with different substrates. In vitro alteration of plasmin, influence of epsilon-aminocaproic acid and tranexamic acid upon its activity.
A: 3.1, S: 7, 12, 13.
Lämmle B, Eichlisberger R, Hänni L, Bounameaux H, Marbet GA, Duckert F: Thrombos Haemostas 42:226, 1979 (Meeting abstract).
Monitoring of oral anticoagulation comparison of the prothrombin time with the colorimetric factor X assay in 107 patients.
A: 2.2, S: 1.
Lämmle B, Eichlisberger R, Hänni L, Bounameaux H, Marbet GA, Duckert F: Schw Med Wo 109:1115–1119, 1979.
Kontrolle der oralen Antikoagulation: Vergleich zwischen quick- und kolori-metrischer Factor-X-Bestimmung bei 107 Patienten. (Control of oral anticoagulation: comparison between quick and colorimetric factor X determination in 107 patients.)
A: 2.2, S: 1.
Lämmle B, Eichlisberger R, Marbet GA, Duckert F: Thromb Res 16:245–254, 1980.
Amidolytic activity in normal human plasma assessed with chromogenic substrates.
A: 7, S: 3, 6, 7, 8, 9, 11, 12, 13, 19.
Lane DA, MacGregor I, Scully MF, Kakkar VV: *In* MF Scully, VV Kakkar (eds). Chromogenic Peptide Substrates: Chemistry and Clinical Usage. Livingstone, London, 1979, pp 206–218.
Use of chromogenic substrates in the study of heparin heterogeneity: influence of platelet and plasma heparin neutralizing activity.
A: 1.3, 2.3, S: 1, 8.

Larsen ML, Abilgaard U, Teien AN, Gjesdal K: Thromb Res 13:285—288, 1978.
Assay of plasma heparin using thrombin and the chromogenic substrate H-D-Phe-Pip-Arg. pNA (S 2238).
A: 1.3, S: 8.

Latallo ZS, Poller R: *In* Advances in Blood Coagulation. Churchill Livingstone, London, in press.
A: 9.

Latallo ZS, Teisseyre E: IXth meeting of the Federation of European Biochemical Societies, Budapest, August 1974 (Meeting abstract).
Preliminary experience with a new chromogenic substrate in studies on blood coagulation and fibrinolysis.
A: 7.

Latallo ZS, Teisseyre E: *In* I Witt (ed). New Methods for the Analysis of Coagulation using Chromogenic Substrates. de Gruyter, Berlin, 1977, pp 181—192.
Amidolytic assay of prothrombin activated with Ecarin, a procoagulant from Echis Carinatus Venom.
A: 1.2, S: 8, 9, 11.

Latallo ZS, Teisseyre E. Lopaciuk S: Thrombos Haemostas 38:21, 1977 (Meeting abstract).
Assessment of plasma fibrinolytic system with chromogenic substrate.
A: 3.1, 3.3, 3.4, S: 12.

Latallo ZS, Teisseyre E, Lopaciuk S: Haemostasis 7: 150—154, 1978.
Assessment of plasma fibrinolytic system with use of chromogenic substrates.
A: 3.1, 3.2, 3.3, 3.4, S: 12.

Latallo ZS, Teisseyre E, Lopaciuk S: *In* MF Scully, VV Kakkar (eds). Chromogenic Peptide Substrates: Chemistry and Clinical Usage. Churchill Livingstone, London, 1979, pp 262—266.
Evaluation of a fibrinolytic profile of plasma using chromogenic substrates.
A: 3.1, 3.2, 3.3, 3.4, S: 12.

Latallo ZS, Teisseyre E, Raczka E: *In* MF Scully, VV Kakkar (eds). Chromogenic Peptide Substrates: Chemistry and Clinical Usage. Churchill Livingstone, London, 1979, pp 154—162.
Activators of plasminogen, measurement using chromogenic substrates.
A: 3.4, S: 12, 13.

Latallo ZS, Thomson JM, Poller L: Br J Haematol 47:307—318, 1981.
An evaluation of chromogenic substrates in the control of oral anticoagulant therapy.
A: 1.2, 2.2, S: 1.

Lawson DE, Mitchell GA, Huseby RM: Thromb Res 14:323—332, 1979.
A sensitive fluorescent assay for determining α_2-plasmin inhibitor using a synthetic substrate.
A: 3.3, S: 16.

Lill H, Roeschlau P, Jilek F, Munz E: Blut 42:132, 1981 (Meeting abstract).
Photometric test for determination of prothrombin in plasma.
A: 1.2, S: 9.

Lindahl U, Kolset SO, Bøgwald J, Østerund B, Seljelid R: Biochem J 206:231—237, 1982.
Studies, with a luminogenic peptide substrate, on blood-coagulation factor-X X_a produced by mouse peritoneal-macrophages.
A: 2.1, 2.2, S: 22.

Lindhout MJ, Kop-Klaasen BHM, Hemker HC: Biochim Biophys Acta 533:342—354, 1978.
The effect of gamma-carboxyglutamate residues on the enzymatic properties of the activated blood clotting factor X. I. Activity towards synthetic substrates.
A: 2.1, S: 1, 11, 17.

Lindhout MJ, Kop-Klaassen BHM, Hemker HC: Biochim Biophys Acta 533:327–341, 1978.
Activation of decarboxyfactor X by a protein from Russell's Viper Venom. Purification and partial characterization of activated decarboxy Factor X.
A: 2.2, S: 1.

Liu HY, Peltz GA, Leytus SP, Livingstone C, Brocklehurst J, Mangel WF: Proc Natl Acad Sci USA 77:3796–3800, 1981.
Sensitive assay for plasminogen activator of transformed cells.
A: 3.4, S: 16.

Long WF, Williams FB, Frazer JD, Scott GK: I.R.C.S.-Bioch 10:208, 1982.
Human leukocyte surface proteinase-catalysed amidolysis is inhibited by anionic polysaccharide modulated antithrombin-III.
A: 7.

Lorand L, Credo RB: In RL Lundblad, JW Fenton, KG Mann (eds). The Chemistry and Biology of Thrombin. Ann Arbor Science Publ inc, Ann Arbor, Mich, 1977, pp 311–323.
Thrombin and fibrinstabilization.
A: 7.

Lottenberg R, Christensen U, Jackson CM, Coleman PL: Meth Enzym 80 (PC):341–361, 1981.
Assay of coagulation proteases using peptide chromogenic and fluorogenic substrates.
A: 7.

Lottenberg R, Hall JA, Fenton JW II, Jackson CM: Thrombosis Reasearch 1982 (in press).
A: 9.

Lottenberg R, Jackson CM: Thrombos Haemostas 46:178, 1981 (Meeting abstract).
Substrate specificity of bovine thrombin and factor X_a toward peptide para-nitroanilide substrates.
A: 7.

Lottenberg R, Jackson CM: Biochim Biophys Acta 1982 (in press).
A: 9.

MacGregor IR, Lane DA, Kakkar VV: Biochim Biophys Acta 586:584–593, 1980.
Evidence for a plasma inhibitor of the heparin accelerated inhibition of factor X_a by antithrombin III.
A: 1.3, 2.3, S: 1, 8.

Mackie IJ, Seghatchian MJ: Thrombos Haemostas 46:314, 1981 (Meeting abstract).
FVIII:C Inhibitor assays by amidolytic methods.
A: 2.4, S: 1.

Mackie M, Booth NA, Bennett B: Br J Haematol 47:77–90, 1981.
Comparative studies on human activators of plasminogen.
A: 3.4, S: 19.

Magnusson S, Sottrup-Jensen L, Petersen TE, Dudek-Wojciechowska G, Claeys H: In DW Ribbon, K Brew (eds). Proteolysis and Physiological Regulation. Academic Press, New York, NY, 1976, pp 203–238.
A: 9.

Margarit P, Deutsch E: Thromb Res 21:585–591, 1981.
Clinical use of a method for the determination of factor VII by a chromogenic substrate.
A: 2.4, S: 1.

Margolius HS, Chao J: J Clin Invest 65:1343–1350, 1981.
Amiloride inhibits mammalian renal kallikrein and a kallikrein-like enzyme from toad bladder and skin.
A: 5.1, S: 17.

Marlar RA, Walz DA, Fenton JW, Seegers WH. American Chemical Society Div Biol Chem 17th National Meeting 1977 (Meeting abstract).
A: 9.

Marossy K, Hauck M, Elödi P: Biochim Biophys Acta 615:237–245, 1981.
Purification and characterization of the elastase-like enzyme of the bovine granulocyte.
A: 6, S: 17.

Mattia D De, Montagna O, Marvulli E: Boll Soc Ital Biol Sper 55:746–750, 1981.
Il dosaggio dell' antithrombina III con substrato cromogenico nell' eta neonatale.
A: 1.3, S: 9.

Mattler LE, Bang NU: Thrombos Haemostas 38:776–792, 1977.
Serine protease specificity for peptide chromogenic substrates.
A: 7.

McKay EJ: Br J Haematol 46:277–285, 1981.
Immunochemical analysis of active and inactive antithrombin III.
A: 1.3, S: 8.

McLellan DS, Devlin JD, Heyse-Moore GH, Aronstam A: J Clin Pathol 33:438–444, 1980.
Comparison of three methods for the estimation of plasma antithrombin.
A: 1.3, S: 8.

McRae BJ, Kurachi K, Heimark RL, Fujikawa K, Davie EW, Powers JC: Biochemistry 20:7196–7206, 1981.
Mapping the active sites of bovine thrombin, factor IX_a, factor X_a, factor XI_a, factor XII_a, plasma kallikrein, and trypsin with amino acid and peptide thioesters: development of new sensitive substrates.
A: 7.

McRae BJ, Nakajima K, Travis J, Powers JC: Biochemistry 19:3973–3978, 1980.
Studies on reactivity of human leukocyte elastase, cathepsin G and porcine pancreatic elastase toward peptides including sequences related to the reactive site of α_1-protease inhibitor (α_1 antitrypsin).
A: 7.

Messmore HL, Fareed J, Gallagher J, Orfei P: Thrombos Haemostas 42:399, 1979 (Meeting abstract).
Inhibition of the amidolytic and procoagulant actions of bovine factor X_a by H-D-Pro-Phe-Arg-NH_2 (S 2443), H-D-Phe-Phe-Arg-NH_2 (S 2448), H-D-Pro-Phe-Arg OH (S 2430) and their derivatives.
A: 7.

Messmore HL, Fareed J, Kniffin J, Squillac G, Walenga J: Ann NY Acad 370:785–797, 1981.
Synthetic substrate assays of the coagulation enzymes and their inhibitors-comparison with clotting and immunological methods for clinical and experimental usage.
A: 1.3, 2.3, 3.2, 3.3, S: 5, 8, 9, 12, 13.

Messmore HL, Fareed J, Walenga JM: Thrombos Haemostas 46:314, 1981 (Meeting abstract).
Problematic aspects of synthetic peptide substrate assays for coagulation parameters.
A: 1.2, 2.2, 3.3, 4.1.

Mibashan RS, Scully MF, Birch AJ, Thumpston JK, MacGregor IB, VV Kakkar: Thrombos Haemostas 42:291, 1979 (Meeting abstract).
Automated control of coumarin therapy by chromogenic factor X assay.
A: 2.2, S: 1.

Milad MP, Hassouna HI: Thrombos Haemostas 46:46, 1981 (Meeting abstract).
Clotting and chromogenic substrate assays measure separate thrombin activities.
A: 1.3, S: 8.

Miller-Andersson M: To be published.
Problems of quantitation of thrombin activity.
A: 9.

Miller-Andersson M, Seghatchian MJ: Proceedings of synthetic substrates and inhibitors of coagulation and fibrinolysis. 22nd Annual Meeting Int Committee on Thrombosis and Haemostasis, Kyoto, 1976, pp 49—50.
Standardization of thrombin using clotting technique and synthetic substrates. Divergency between different standards.
A: 1.1.

Miller-Andersson M, Seghatchian MJ: Thrombos Haemostas 38:162, 1977 (Meeting abstract).
In vitro thrombogenicity test for clinical factor IX concentrates using synthetic substrates.
A: 7.

Miller-Andersson M, Seghatchian J: Haemostasis 7:113—120, 1978.
Microheterogeneity in thrombin standards.
A: 1.1, S: 1, 8, 9, 11, 12.

Mitchell GA, Abdullah CM, Ruiz JA, Huseby RM, Alvarez de Geiger TM, Black FM, Heller ZH: Thromb Res 21:573—584, 1981.
Fluorogenic substrate assays for factor VIII and factor IX — Introduction of a new solid-phase fluorescent detection method.
A: 1.4, S: 16.

Mitchell GA, Gargiulo RJ, Huseby RM, Lawson DE, Pochron SP, Sehuanes JA: Thromb Res 13:47—52, 1979.
Assay for plasma heparin using a synthetic peptide substrate for thrombin. Introduction of the fluorophore aminoisophthalic acid, dimethyl ester.
A: 1.3, S: 16.

Mitchell GA, Hudson PM, Huseby RM, Pochron SP, Gargiulo RJ: Thromb Res 12: 219—225, 1978.
Fluorescent substrate assay for antithrombin III.
A: 1.3, S: 16.

Morita T, Kato H, Iwanaga S, Takada K, Kimura T, Sakakibara S: J Biochem (Tokyo) 82:1495—1498, 1978.
New fluorogenic substrates for α-thrombin, factor X_a, kallikreins, and urokinase.
A: 1.1, 2.1, 3.4, 4.1, S: 16.

Morisson-Silverberg SA, Jesty J: J Biol Chem 256:1625—1630, 1981.
The role of activated factor X in the control of bovine coagulation factor VII.
A: 2.1, S: 1.

Mussoni L, Raczka E, Chmielewska J, Donati MB, Latallo ZS: Thromb Res 15:341— 349, 1979.
Plasminogen assay in rabbit, rat and mouse plasma using the chromogenic substrate S 2251.
A: 3.2, S: 12.

Naito K, Aoki N: Thromb Res 12:1147—1156, 1978.
Assay of α_2-plasmin inhibitor activity by means of a plasmin specific tripeptide substrate.
A: 3.3, S: 12.

Nakamura S, Morita T, Iwanaga S, Niwa M, Takahashi T: J Biochem 81:1567—1569, 1977.
A sensitive substrate for the clotting enzyme in horseshoe crab hemocytes.
A: 5.3, S: 1.

Nakamura S, Morita T, Harada-Suzuki T, Iwanaga S, Takahashi K, Niwa M: J Biochem 92:781—792, 1982.

A clotting enzyme associated with the hemolymph coagulation system of horseshoe crab (*Tachypleus tridentatus*): Its purification and characterization.
A: 7, S: 19.

Nakamura S, Takizawa N, Nakanishi K, Igarashi M: Rinsho Byori 28:670–674, 1981 (author's transl.)
On the determination of plasma prekallikrein with chromogenic peptide substrate.
A: 4.1, S: 6.

Nenci GG, Berrettini M, Agnelli G, Parise P: Boll Soc Ital Biol Sper 56:519–525, 1980.
Heparin assay: a comparison between titrimetric and amidolytic methods.
A: 2.3, S: 1.

Nienhaus Kh, Jäger H, Wenzel E, Pfordt L, Taubert W, Hellstern P: 1. Blut 40:54, 1980 (Meeting abstract).
Spezifität und Aussagekraft amidolytisch-fotometrischer, immunologischer und konventionell-gerinnungsphysiologischer Laborparameter zur Verlaufskontrolle der fibrinolytischen Therapie.
A: 7.

Nienhaus Kh, Wenzel E, Jäger H, Pfordt L, Biemer I: Thrombos Haemostas 42:50, 1979 (Meeting abstract).
Photometric measurement of fibrinolytic activities during urokinase therapy.
A: 3.1, 3.4, S: 4, 13, 19.

Nieuwenhuizen W, Wijngaards G, Groeneveld E: Anal Biochemistry 83:143–148, 1977.
Fluorogenic peptide amide substrates for the estimation of plasminogen activators and plasmin.
A: 3.1, 3.4, S: 16.

Nieuwenhuizen W, Wijngaards G, Groeneveld E: Thrombos Haemostas 38:21, 1977 (Meeting abstract).
Fluorogenic substrates for the determination of plasminogen activators and plasmin.
A: 3.1, 3.4, S: 16.

Nieuwenhuizen W, Wijngaards G, Groeneveld E: Thromb Res 11:87–89, 1977.
Synthetic substrates and the discrimination between urokinase and tissue plasminogen activator activity.
A: 3.4, S: 16.

Nieuwenhuizen W, Wijngaards G, Groeneveld E: Haemostasis 7:146–149, 1978.
Fluorogenic substrates for sensitive and differential estimation of urokinase and tissue plasminogen activator.
A: 3.4, S: 16.

Nigretto JM, Jozefowics M: Thromb Res 17:611–622, 1980.
The electrochemical activity determination of trypsin-like enzymes I. Trypsin.
A: 6, S: 20.

Niinobe M, Hitomi Y, Fujii S: J Biochem (Tokyo) 87:779–783, 1980.
A sensitive colorimetric assay for various proteases using naphthyl ester derivatives as substrates.
A: 1.1, 3.1, 3.4, S: 17.

Nishibe H: Clin Chim Acta 106:301–307, 1981.
The assay of factor V in plasma using a synthetic chromogenic substrate.
A: 1.5, S: 8.

Nijman D, Duckert F: Thromb Diath Haemorrh 33:221–225, 1975.
Assay of brinase inhibitors with soluble and insoluble substrates.
A: 6, S: 11.

O'Brien PF: Thrombos Haemostas 43:69, 1980.
The chromogenic assay of low levels of heparin in plasma: Probable effect of platelets.
A: 2.3, S: 1.

154

O'Brien PF: Thrombos Haemostas 46:383, 1981 (Meeting abstract).
Fluorometric assay of low-dose plasma heparin.
A: 1.3, S: 16.

O'Brien PF, Clemenson J, Browse NL: Thrombos Haemostas 46:381, 1981 (Meeting abstract).
Plasma heparin and antithrombin III response following endotracheal administration of heparin.
A: 9.

Ødegard OR: Thromb Res 7:351–360, 1975.
Evaluation of an amidolytic heparin cofactor assay method.
A: 1.3, S: 11.

Ødegard OR, Abildgaard U: *In* I Witt (ed). New Methods for the Analysis of Coagulation using Chromogenic Substrates. de Gruyter, Berlin, 1977, pp 123–129.
Determination of antithrombin III and antifactor X_a activity.
A: 1.3, 2.3, S: 1, 8, 11.

Ødegard OR, Abildgaard U: Haemostasis 7:127–134, 1978.
Antithrombin III: Critical review of assay methods.
A: 1.3, 2.3, S: 1, 8, 9, 11.

Ødegard OR, Abildgaard U, Lie M, Miller-Andersson M: Thromb Res 11:205–216, 1977.
Inactivation of bovine and human thrombin and factor X_a by antithrombin III studied with amidolytic methods.
A: 1.3, 2.3, S: 1, 8, 11.

Ødegard OR, Lie M: Haemostasis 7:121–126, 1978.
On use of chromogenic substrates for studies of coagulation inhibitors.
A: 1.3, 2.3, S: 1, 8, 9.

Ødegard OR, Lie M, Abildgaard U: Thromb Res 6:287–294, 1975.
Heparin cofactor activity measured with an amidolytic method.
A: 1.3, S: 11.

Ødegard OR, Lie M, Abildgaard U: Haemostasis 5:265–275, 1976.
Antifactor X_a activity measured with amidolytic methods.
A: 2.3, S: 1.

Ødegard OR, Rosenlund B, Ervik E: Haemostasis 7:202–209, 1978.
Automated antithrombin III assay with a centrifugal analyser.
A: 2.3, S: 1.

Oguma Y, Seya T, Murakoshi T, Yamauchi M, Nagata H, Hasgawa H: Thrombos Haemostas 42:379, 1979 (Meeting abstract).
Assay of heparin in plasma using a chromogenic substrate and its clinical applications.
A: 9.

Oh-ishi S, Katori M: Thromb Res 14:551–559, 1979.
Fluorometric assay for plasma prekallikrein using peptidylmethyl-coumarinyl-amide as a substrate.
A: 4.1, S: 16.

Ohno Y, Kato H, Iwanaga S, Takada K, Sakakibara S, Stenflo J: The 100th Congress on Japanese Pharmaceutical Society (Tokyo) 1980 (Meeting abstract).
A new fluorogenic peptide substrate for blood coagulation factor, protein C.
A: 6, S: 16.

Ohno Y, Kato H, Morita T, Iwanaga S, Takada K, Sakakibara S, Stenflo J: J Biochem 90:1387–1395, 1981.
A new fluorogenic peptide substrate for vitamin K-dependent blood coagulation factor, bovine protein-C.
A: 6, S: 16.

Ohno H, Kosaki G, Kambayashi J, Imaoka S, Hirata F: Thromb Res 19:579–588, 1981.

(Ethyl P-(6-guanidinohexanoyloxy) Benzoate) methanesulfonate as a serine proteinase inhibitor. I. Inhibition of thrombin and factor X_a in vitro.
A: 1.1, 2.1, 3.1, 4.1, 5.1, S: 1, 5, 7, 8, 12.
Oka K, Tanaka K: Thromb Res 19:125−128, 1980.
Histochemical demonstration of thrombin using fluorogenic substrate.
A: 1.1, S: 16, 21.
Okamoto S, Ikezawa K, Nagano S, Matsuoka A, Hijikato A, Tamao Y: Thrombos Haemostas 46:313, 1981 (Meeting abstract).
Selectivity increase of chromogenic assay of factor X_a by use of highly selective synthetic thrombin inhibitor having extremely potent stereostructure (No. 805).
A: 2.1, S: 1.
Okamoto U, Nagamatsu Y, Horie N, Okada Y, Tsuda Y: Thrombos Haemostas 46:86, 1981 (Meeting abstract).
New synthetic peptide substrates of -Val-pNA type for an insoluble fibrinolytic serine enzyme extracted from human spleen.
A: 6, S: 19.
Okamoto U, Nagamatsu Y, Tsuda Y, Okada Y: Bioc Biop R 97:28−32, 1980.
A new polypeptide substrate suc-Tyr-Leu-Val-pNA, specific for spleen fibrinolytic proteinase (SFP).
A: 6, S: 19.
Oostrijck R: Thrombos Haemostas 42:442, 1979 (Meeting abstract).
Three sources of purified factor III for monitoring vitamin K-dependent coagulation factors using a synthetic chromogenic substrate.
A: 8, S: 8.
Orthner CL, Kosow DD: Arch Biochem Biophys 185:400−406, 1978.
The effect of metal ions on the amidolytic activity of human factor X_a (activated Stuart-Prower Factor).
A: 2.1, S: 1.
Orthner CL, Morris S, Kosov DP: Thromb Res 23:533−539, 1981.
Inhibition of human coagulation factor-X_a by thrombin substrates.
A: 7, S: 1, 8, 11.

Paar D, Maruhn D: J Clin Chem Clin Biochem 18:557−562, 1981.
Spectrometric determination of urokinase in urine after gel filtration, using the chromogenic substrate S 2444.
A: 3.4, S: 3.
Palkuti HS: Am J Med TE 48:109−116, 1982.
Hemostasis. 2. Investigation of the coagulation-factors by use of qualitative and quantitative assay techniques.
A: 7.
Parvez Z, Fareed J, Messmore HL, Moncada R: Fed Proc 41:1122, 1982 (Meeting abstract).
Non linearity of amidolytic assays for functional antithrombin-III (AT-III) quantitation in clinical samples and reference plasmas.
A: 7.
Paulssen MMP, Kolhorn A, Rothuizen J, Planje MC: Clin Chim A 92:465−468, 1979.
Automated amidolytic assay of thrombin generation − alternative for the prothrombin-time test.
A: 8, S: 9.
Perry JF, Wehrly JA, Coleman PL: Thrombos Haemostas 46:374, 1981 (Meeting abstract).
Application of enzyme kinetic analysis in the development of an automated antithrombin III assay.
A: 1.3.

156

Philo RD, Gaffney PJ: Thrombos Haemostas 46:375, 1981 (Meeting abstract).
The effects of defibrination procedures in plasma ATIII assays.
A: 1.3, S: 8.
Philo RD, Gaffney PJ: Br J Haem 50:147–156, 1982.
Comparison of antithrombin-III assays using biological and chromogenic substrates.
A: 1.3, S: 8.
Pierzchala PA, Dorn CP, Zimmerman M: Biochem J 183:555–559, 1979.
A new fluorogenic substrate for plasmin.
A: 3.1, S: 16.
Pindur G, Seifried E, Joos A, Rasche H: Med Lab (Stuttg.) 34:88–91, 1981.
Gerinnungsüberwachung der oralen Antikoagulantien Therapie unter Verwendung chromogener Substrate.
A: 1.2, 2.2, S: 1, 8.
Plaut GWE: Haemostasis 7:105–108, 1978.
p-Nitrobenzyl-p-Toluenesulfonyl-L-Arginine: a chromogenic substrate for thrombin, plasmin and trypsin.
A: 1.1, 3.1, 6, S: 17.
Pochron SP, Mitchell GA, Albareda I, Huseby RM, Cargiulo RJ: Thromb Res 13:733–739, 1978.
A fluorescent substrate assay for plasminogen.
A: 3.2, S: 16.
Poggi M, Palareti G, Coccheri S: Thrombos Haemostas 46:372, 1981 (Meeting abstract).
A comparison of various methods for measuring AT III in different clinical conditions.
A: 7, S: 8.
Pogliani EM, Vigo A, Cofrancesco E, Colombi M, Critoforetti, G, Marchetti G, Vercesi G, Radaelli F: Thromb Res 27:211–219, 1982.
Low-dose heparin in thoracic-surgery-effect on blood coagulation and fibrinolysis system.
A: 1.3, 2.3, 3.3, 4.1, S: 1, 7, 8, 12.
Poller L, Latallo ZS: Brit J Haem 50:688, 1982 (Meeting abstract).
An assessment of an amidolytic assay for factor VII in the laboratory control of oral anticoagulants.
A: 2.4, S; 2.
Poller L, Thomson JM, Bodzenta A, Easton AC, Latallo ZS, Chmielewska J: Br J Haem 49:69–75, 1981.
An assessment of an amidolytic assay for factor VII in the laboratory control of oral anticoagulants.
A: 2.4, S: 2.
Potron G, LaFaurie M, Droulle C: Thrombos Haemostas 46:363, 1981 (Meeting abstract).
Application of enzymatic methods on chromogen substrates in animals compared coagulation.
A: 1.3, 2.1, 3.1, 3.3, 4.1, S: 1, 7, 9, 12.
Potron G, Lafaurie M, Remy MG, Florent B, Droulle C: Nouv Rf Hem 22:297–298, 1980.
Application of enzyme methods to chromogenous substrates in comparative clotting.
A: 7.
Powers JC, McRae BJ: Thrombos Haemostas 46:327, 1981 (Meeting abstract).
Amino acid and peptide thioesters: new sensitive substrates for bovine factors IX_a, X_a, XI_a, XII_a, thrombin, plasma kallikrein and trypsin.
A: 7, S: 18.

Pozsgay M, Gáspár R Jr, Elödi P, Bajusz S: FEBS letters 74:67–70, 1977.
Investigations on new tripeptidyl-p-nitroanilide substrates for subtilisins.
A: 6, S: 11, 12, 19.

Pozsgay M, Szabo G, Bajusz S, Simonsson R, Gaspar R, Elödi P: Eur J Biochem 115:491–495, 1981.
Studies of the specificity of thrombin with tripeptidyl-p-nitroanilide substrates.
A: 7.

Putten JJ van, Ruit M van de, Beunis M, Hemker HC: Clin Chem Acta 122:261–270, 1982.
Interindividual variation in relationships between plasma heparin concentration and the results of fine heparin assays.
A: 2.3, S: 1.

Ratnoff OD: J Lab Clin Med 96:267–277, 1980.
The relative amidolytic activity of Hageman factor (factor XII) and its fragments. The effect of high-molecular-weight kininogen and kaolin.
A: 4.2, S: 8.

Ratnoff OD: Blood 57:55–58, 1981.
Studies on the inhibition of ellagic acid-activated Hageman factor (factor XII) and Hageman factor fragments.
A: 4.2, S: 8.

Reiter B, Tiesler E, Pfordt L, Wenzel E, Nienhaus Kh, Hellstern P: Blut 40:97, 1980 (Meeting abstract).
Nachweis von Streptokinase-ähnlichen Aktivitäten in A-Streptokokken mittels fotometrischer Analyse unter Verwendung chromogener Substrate.
A: 3.4, S: 3, 13.

Risberg B, Claeson G: In JF Davidson (ed). Progress in chemical fibrinolysis and thrombolysis Vol. IV. Churchill Livingstone, London, 1979, pp 164–166.
A new quantitative method for determination of plasminogen tissue activators.
A: 3.4, S: 19.

Robbins KC, Wohl RC, Summaria L: Haemostasis 7:137, 1978.
Catalytic efficiency of activation of human plasminogen by various activator species.
A: 3.4, S: 12.

Róka L, Bleyl H: In I Witt (ed). New Methods for the Analysis of Coagulation using Chromogenic Substrates. de Gruyter, Berlin, 1977, pp 105–116.
Studies on the determination of anti-thrombin.
A: 1.3, S: 11.

Róka L, Bleyl H: In MF Scully, VV Kakkar (eds). Chromogenic Peptide Substrates: Chemistry and Clinical Usage. Churchill Livingstone, London, 1979, pp 192–195.
Experiences with the determination of antithrombin III, heparin and prothrombin with chromozym TH.
A: 1.2, 1.3, S: 9.

Róka L, Koch R, Bleyl H: In I Witt (ed). New Methods for the Analysis of Coagulation using Chromogenic Substrates. de Gruyter, Berlin, 1977, pp 171–180.
Studies on the determination of prothrombin with S 2160.
A: 1.2, S: 11.

Róka L, Rasche H: Internist (Berlin) 21:189–194, 1981.
Blutgerinnungskiagnostik mit chromogenen Substraten.
A: 7.

Rosing J, Tans G, Govers-Riemslag JWP, Zwaal RFA, Hemker HC: J Biol Chem 255: 274–283, 1980.
The role of phospholipids and factor V_a in the prothrombinase complex.
A: 7, S: 1, 8.

Roth M, Haarsma M: *In* I Witt (ed). New Methods for the Analysis of Coagulation using Chromogenic Substrates. de Gruyter, Berlin, 1977, pp 91–103.
Enzymatic determination of thrombin and thrombin inhibitors.
A: 1.2, 1.3, S: 9, 11.
Rutllant ML: Sangre 23:858–863, 1978.
Papel de los substratos cromogénicos en el estudio de la coagulación y la fibrinólisis.
A: 7.
Rybák M, Simonianová E, Rybákova B, Loštický C: *In* JF Davidson (ed). Progress in Chemical Fibrinolysis and Thrombolysis Vol. IV. Churchill Livingstone, London, 1979, pp 171–173.
The application of amidic substrates for plasmin, thrombin and kallikrein to the study of some problems in fibrinolysis and coagulation.
A: 7, S: 6, 9, 13, 19.

Samama M, Schlegel N, Cazanave B, Horellou MH, Conard J, Castel M, Douenias R: *In* HR Lijnen, D Collen M Verstraete (eds). Synthetic Substrates in Clinical Blood Coagulation Assays. Martinus Nijhoff Publishers, The Hague, 1980, pp 93–98.
α_2-Antiplasmin assay: amidolytic and immunological method. Critical evaluation. Results in a clinical material.
A: 3.3, S: 12.
Sampaio MU, Galembeck F, Paiva AC, Prado ES: Gen Pharmacol 7:167–171, 1976.
Kinetics of the hydrolysis of synthetic substrates by horse urinary kallikrein and trypsin.
A: 7, S: 17, 19.
Sandberg H, Andersson LO: Thromb Res 14:113–124, 1979.
A highly sensitive assay of platelet factor 3 using a chromogenic substrate.
A: 1.4, S: 8.
Sandberg H, Gellerbring AK, Andersson LO: Thrombos Haemostas 42:55, 1979, (Meeting abstract).
Levels of platelet factor 3 in citrate plasma and in whole blood as determined by a chromogenic peptide substrate assay.
A: 1.4, S: 8.
Sandberg H, Gellerbring AK, Andersson LO: Thromb Res 18:871–882, 1980.
Determination of platelet factor 3 in whole blood by a chromogenic peptide substrate assay.
A: 1.4, S: 8.
Sandjberg Hansen M, Clemmensen I: Biochem J 187:173–180, 1980.
Partial purification and characterization of a new fast-acting plasmin inhibitor from human platelets. Evidence for non-identity with the known plasma proteinase inhibitors.
A: 3.3, S: 12.
Sandjberg Hansen M, Petersen LChr: Thrombos Haemostas 46:388, 1981 (Meeting abstract).
Kinetic characterization of the fast acting plasmin inhibitor from human platelets.
A: 3.3, S: 12.
Schöndorf TH, Lasch HG: *In* HR Lijnen, D Collen, M Verstraete (eds). Synthetic Substrates in Clinical Blood Coagulation Assays. Martinus Nijhoff Publishers, The Hague, 1980, pp 51–57.
Antithrombin III and factor X_a determination in patients with low dose heparin and hip surgery.
A: 1.3, S: 8, 9.
Scriban R, Hébert JP, Devillers G: Bios 4:42–48, 1976.
Etude d'un nouveau substrat chromogéne pour la recherche et le dosage des enzymes protéolytiques: LS-2160 de chez Bofors.
A: 7, S: 11.

Scully MF, Kakkar VV: Clin Chimica Acta 79:595–602, 1977.
  Semi micro or automated determination of thrombin, antithrombin and heparin
  cofactor using the substrate, H-D-Phe-Pip-Arg-p-Nitroanilide, 2HCl.
  A: 1.1, 1.3, S: 8.
Scully MF, Kakkar VV: Thromb Res 12:1201–1205, 1978.
  Method for the determination of plasminogen which discriminates between native
  and degraded plasminogen.
  A: 3.2, S: 12.
Scully MF, Kakkar VV: Thrombos Haemostas 42:294, 1979 (Meeting abstract).
  Measurement of native and degraded forms of plasminogen in human plasma.
  A: 3.2, S: 12.
Scully MF, Kakkar VV: In MF Scully, VV Kakkar (eds). Chromogenic Peptide Sub-
  strates: Chemistry and Clinical Usage. Churchill Livingstone, London, 1979, pp
  141–153.
  Measurements of levels of degraded plasminogen during thrombolytic therapy.
  A: 3.2, S: 12.
Scully MF, Mibashan RS, Birch ADJ, Thumpston JK, McGregor IR, North WRS,
  Kakkar VV: In HR Lijnen, D Collen, M Verstraete (eds). Synthetic Substrates
  in Clinical Blood Coagulation Assays. Martinus Nijhoff Publishers, The Hague,
  1980, pp 27–31.
  Automated control of coumarin therapy by chromogenic factor X assay.
  A: 2.2 S: 1.
Searls DB: Anal Biochem 107:64–70, 1981.
  An improved colorimetric assay for plasminogen activator.
  A: 3.4, S: 12.
Seghatchian MJ: In Proceedings of synthetic substrates and inhibitors of coagulation
  and fibrinolysis. 22nd Annual Meeting of the International Committee on Throm-
  bosis and Haemostasis. Kyoto, 1976, pp 49–50.
  A: 9.
Seghatchian MJ: Med Lab Sciences 35:343–346, 1978.
  A new approach to the determination of coagulation factors using chromogenic
  substrates.
  A: 1.1, 2.4, 8, S. 1, 8, 11.
Seghatchian MJ: Thrombos Haemostas 42:111, 1979 (Meeting abstract).
  Electrophoretic distribution of FVIII:C measured by chromogenic and clotting
  methods and comparison with other FVIII-associated activities.
  A: 2.6.
Seghatchian MJ: Thrombos Haemostas 42:238, 1979 (Meeting abstract).
  A tentative cause of discrepancy between FVIII:C estimation.
  A: 7.
Seghatchian MJ: In MF Scully, VV Kakkar (eds). Chromogenic Peptide Substrates:
  Chemistry and Clinical Usage. Churchill Livingstone, London, 1979, pp 102–116.
  The usefulness of chromogenic substrates in the diagnosis of haemophilia and
  control of blood products.
  A: 2.6, 8, S: 1, 11.
Seghatchian MJ: Ric Clin Lab 11:11–25, 1981.
  The values of synthetic substrates in the improvement of diagnostic tests for
  haemostatic function.
  A: 7.
Seghatchian MJ, Miller-Andersson M: Proceedings of synthetic substrates and inhibi-
  tors of coagulation and fibrinolysis, 22nd Annual meeting International Committee
  on Thrombosis and Haemostasis, Kyoto, 1976, pp 51–53.
  Synthetic substrates as a probe for the detection of trace proteolytic contaminants
  in various blood products.
  A: 7.

160

Seghatchian MJ, Miller-Andersson M: Proceedings of Synthetic Substrates and Inhibitors of Coagulations and Fibrinogen. 22nd Annual Meeting of the International Committee on Thrombosis and Haemostasis, Kyoto, 1976, pp 53–54.
Assay of FVIII using chromogenic substrate.
A: 2.6.
Seghatchian MJ, Miller-Andersson M: Med Lab Sciences 35:347–354, 1978.
A colorimetric evaluation of factor VIII:C Potency.
A: 2.6, S: 1.
Seghatchian MJ, Miller-Andersson M: In Proceedings of the VIth Congr of the World Federation of Haemophilia pp 309–311.
A new sensitive and simple technique for screening FVIII level in blood donors and for detection of haemophilia.
A: 2.6.
Seligsohn U, Østerud R, Rapaport SI: Blood 52:978–988, 1978.
Coupled amidolytic assay for factor VII – Its use with a clotting assay to determine activity state of factor VII.
A: 2.4, S: 1.
Seljelid R, Bäckström G, Lindahl U: Exp Cell Res 129:478–481, 1980.
Proteinase activity in macrophage cultures. Effects of heparin and antithrombin.
A: 7, S: 1, 11.
Shimada H, Mori T, Takada A, Takada Y, Nodo Y, Takai I, Kohda H, Nishimura T: Thrombos Haemostas 46:507–510, 1981.
Use of chromogenic substrate S 2251 for determination of plasminogen activator in rat ovaries.
A: 3.4, S: 12.
Silverberg M, Dunn JT, Garen L, Kaplan AP: J Biol Chem 255:7281–7286, 1980.
Autoactivation of human Hageman factor. Demonstration utilizing a synthetic substrate.
A: 4.2, S: 7.
Simonsson R, Arielly S, Friberger P, Aurell L: Thrombos Haemostas 46:313, 1981 (Meeting abstract).
Chromogenic substrates for granulocyte elastase, chymotrypsin and the subcomponents of CI-esterase.
A: 6, S: 19.
Smith RE, Bissell ER, Mitchell AR, Pearson KW: Thromb Res 17:393–402, 1980.
Direct photometric or fluorometric assay of proteinases using substrates containing 7-amino-4-trifluoromethylcoumarin.
A: 3.1, 6, S: 16.
Smith-Erichsen N, Aasen AO, Amundsen E: Thrombos Haemostas 46:342, 1981 (Meeting abstract).
Use of chromogenic peptide substrate assays in the evaluation of surgical treatment of intra-abdominal sepsis.
A: 1.3, 2.3, 3.2, 3.3, 4.1.
Snape TJ, Griffith D, Vallet L, Wesley ED: Dev Biol Stand 44:115–120, 1980.
The assay of prekallikrein activator in human blood products.
A: 4.1, S: 7.
Somorin O, Tokura S: Biochem SSR 45:887–894, 1980.
Comparative activity of plasmin, thrombin and trypsin on chromogenic arginine-para-nitroanalides.
A: 7.
Soria C, Soria J, Samama M: Pathol Biol Fr 24:725–729, 1976.
Dosage du plasminogène à l'aide d'un substrat chromogène tripeptidique.
A: 3.2, S: 12.
Soria J, Soria C, Boisseau MR, Hourdille P, Sanchez C: In MF Scully, VV Kakkar (eds). Chromogenic Peptide Substrates: Chemistry and Clinical Usage. Churchill Livingstone, London, 1979, pp 93–101.

Measurements of prekallikrein. Clinical application to patients suffering from burns and the relationship between platelet nucleotides and prekallikrine level.
A: 4.1, S: 6.

Soria J, Soria C, Samama M: *In* JF Davidson, RM Rowan, MM Samama, PC Desnoyers (eds). Progress in Chemical Fibrinolysis and Throbolysis 3. Raven Press, New York, 1978, pp 337–346.
A plasminogen assay using a chromogenic synthetic substrate. Results from clinical work and from studies of thrombolysis.
A: 3.2, S: 12.

Sottrup-Jensen L, Claeys H, Zajdel M, Petersen TE, Magnusson S: *In* JF Davidson, RM Rowan, MM Samama, PC Desnoyers (eds). Progress in Chemical Fibrinolysis and Thrombolysis 3. Raven Press, New York, 1978, pp 191–209.
A: 9.

Soulier JP, Gorin D: Thrombos Haemostas 42:538–547, 1979.
Assay of Fletcher factor (plasma prekallikrein) using an artificial clotting reagent and a modified chromogenic assay.
A: 4.1, S: 6.

Stormorken H: Thrombos Haemostas 36:299–301, 1976.
A new era in the laboratory evaluation of coagulation and fibrinolysis. Editorial.
A: 7.

Stormorken H: *In* I Witt (ed). New Methods for the Analysis of Coagulation using Chromogenic Substrates. de Gruyter, Berlin, 1977, pp 119–212.
Studies on antithrombin III using chromozyme TH.
A: 1.3, S: 9.

Stormorken H: *In* MF Scully, VV Kakkar (eds). Chromogenic Peptide Substrates. Chemistry and Clinical Usage. Churchill Livingstone, London, 1979, pp 32–39.
Advantages and disadvantages of assaying coagulation and fibrinolytic parameters using chromogenic substrates.
A: 7.

Stormorken H, Baklund A, Gallimore M, Rilaund S: Haemostasis 7:69–75, 1978.
Chromogenic substrate assay of plasma prekallikrein with a note on its site of biosynthesis.
A: 4.1, S: 6.

Stürzebecher J, Markwardt F, Wagner G, Voigt B: Thromb Res 26:221–226, 1982.
Are synthetic inhibitors able to improve factor X_a assays using peptide substrates?
A: 7.

Sugo T, Hamaguchi A, Shimada T, Kato H, Iwanaga S: J Biochem 92:689–698, 1982.
Mechanism of surface-mediated activation of bovine factor XII and plasma prekallikrein.
A: 7, S: 16.

Sugo T, Ikari N, Kato H, Iwanaga S, Fuji S: Seikagaku S: (in Japanese) 51:589, 1979.
Mechanism of kaolin-mediated activation of Factor XII.
A: 9.

Suomela H: Haemostasis 7:95–96, 1978.
Study of specificity of synthetic substrates in blood coagulation.
A: 7, S: 1, 11, 12, 19.

Suomela H, Blombäck M, Blombäck B: Thromb Res 10:267–281, 1977.
The activation of factor X evaluated by using synthetic substrates.
A: 2.4, S: 1.

Suomela H, Hekali R, Vahvaselkä E: Develop Biol Standard 44:99–105, 1979.
Stability of IgG Solutions, especially anti-D gammaglobulin, with special reference to measured proteolytic activity and degradation.
A: 6, S: 12.

Suzuki K, Nishioka J, Hashimoto S: Rinsho Byori 27:218–222, 1979 (Author's translation).

Assay method for urinary urokinase using synthetic fluorogenic substrate.
A: 3.4, S: 16.
Suzuki K, Nishioka J, Hashimoto S: Rinsho Byori 28:804–807, 1981 (Author's translation).
Assay method of plasma plasminogen by means of a synthetic fluorogenic peptide substrate (3104-V).
A: 3.2, S: 16.
Svendsen L: Aktuelle Diagnostik, Boehringer Mannheim, 1976.
Aktivitätsbestimmung proteolytischer Enzyme mit synthetishen Substraten.
A: 7.
Svendsen L: In I Witt (ed). New Methods for the Analysis of Coagulation using Chromogen Substrates. de Gruyter, Berlin, 1977, pp 251–259.
Estimation of urokinase activity by means of a highly susceptible synthetic chromogenic peptide substrate.
A: 3.4, S: 4.
Svendsen L: In MF Scully, VV Kakkar (eds). Chromogenic Peptide Substrates: Chemistry and Clinical Usage. Churchill Livingstone, London, 1979, pp 13–19.
The use of chromogenic substrates at present and in the future for factors of the coagulation fibrinolytic and kallikrein-kinin systems.
A: 7.
Svendsen L, Amundsen E: IVth Int Congr Thromb Haem, Vienna, 1973 (Meeting abstract).
Estimation of plasmin and Brinase B activities by means of a highly susceptible synthetic chromogenic peptide substrate.
A: 3.1, 6.
Svendsen L, Blombäck B, Blombäck M, Olsson PI: Thromb Res 1:267–278, 1972.
Synthetic chromogenic substrates for determination of trypsin, thrombin, and thrombin-like enzymes.
A: 7, S: 11.
Svendsen L, Stocker K: In I Witt (ed). New Methods for the Analysis of Coagulation using Chromogenic Substrates. de Gruyter, Berlin, 1977, pp 23–35.
Determination of protease activities with specifically constructed peptide-p-nitroanilide derivatives.
A: 7.

Takada A, Ito T, Takada Y: Thrombos Haemostas 43:20–23, 1980.
Interaction of plasmin with tranexamic acid and alpha$_2$ plasmin inhibitor in the plasma clot.
A: 3.4, S: 12.
Takada K, Sakakiba S, Kato H, Goto I, Iwanaga S: Thromb Res 20:533–542, 1980.
Synthesis of Bz-Phe(p-NO$_2$)-Val-Arg-pNA and its specificity to thrombin-like enzymes – similarity of a commercial products S 2160 to the nitrated compound.
A: 7, S: 11.
Takada A, Urano T, Takada Y: Thromb Haemostas 42:901–908, 1979.
Influence of coagulation on the activation of plasminogen by streptokinase and urokinase.
A: 3.4, S: 12.
Takagi K, Moriya A, Tamura H, Nakahara C, Tanaka S, Fujita Y, Kawai T: Thromb Res 23:51–58, 1981.
Quantitative measurement of endotoxin in human blood using synthetic chromogenic substrate for horseshoe crab clotting enzyme: A comparison of methods of blood sampling and treatment.
A: 5.3, S: 19.

Takasaki S, Kasai K, Ishii S: J Biochem 78:1275–1285, 1975.
Comparison of the catalytic properties of thrombin and trypsin by kinetic analysis on the basis of active enzyme concentration.
A: 7, S: 17.
Tamura H, Obayashi T, Takagi K, Tanaka S, Nakakara C, Kawai T: Thromb Res 27: 51–52, 1982.
Perchloric-acid treatment of human-blood for quantitative endotoxin assay using synthetic chromogenic substrate for Horseshoe crab clotting enzyme.
A: 5.3, S: 19.
Tankersley KL, Alving BM, Finlayson JS: Thrombos Haemostas 46:231, 1981 (Meeting abstract).
Activation of factor XII by dextran sulfate: a convenient assay for factor XII.
A: 7, S: 7.
Tans G, Janssen-Claessen T, Dieijen G van, Rosing J, Hemker HC: Thrombos Haemostas 46:256, 1981 (Meeting abstract).
Activation of bovine factor IX by bovine factor XI_a. Active site titration of factor IX_a and development of a spectrophotometric assay for factor IX.
A: 2.4, S: 1.
Teger-Nilsson AC: In MF Scully, VV Kakkar (eds). Chromogenic Peptide Substrates: Chemistry and Clinical Usage. Churchill Livingstone, London, 1979, pp 269–276.
Use of chromogenic substrates for screening of inhibitors of coagulation and fibrinolysis in patients.
A: 3.1, 3.3, S: 8, 11, 12.
Teger-Nilsson AC, Friberger P, Gyzander E: Scand J Clin Lab Invest 37:403–409, 1977.
Determination of a new rapid plasmin inhibitor in human blood by means of a specific tripeptide substrate.
A: 3.3, S: 12.
Teger-Nilsson AC, Friberger P, Gyzander E: In JF Davidson, RM Rowan, MM Samama, P Desnoyers (eds). Progress in Chemical Fibrinolysis and Thrombolysis 3. Raven Press, New York, 1978, pp 305–313.
Antiplasmin determination by means of a chromogenic tripeptide substrate.
A: 3.3, S: 12.
Teger-Nilsson AC, Gyzander E, Hedner U, Myrwold H, Nappa H, Olsson R, Wallmo L: In JF Davidson, RM Rowan, MM Samama, PC Desnoyers (eds). Progress in Chemical Fibrinolysis and Thrombolysis Vol. 3. Raven Press, New York, 1978, pp 327–335.
Antiplasmin and other natural inhibitors of fibrinolysis in clinical material.
A: 3.3, S: 12.
Teien AN: In MF Scully, VV Kakkar (eds). Chromogenic Peptide Substrates: Chemistry and Clinical Usage. Churchill Livingstone, London, 1979, pp 196–204.
Assay of heparin using Factor X_a and a chromogenic substrate.
A: 2.3, S: 1.
Teien AN, Abildgaard U, Hook M, Lindahl U: Thromb Res 11:107–117, 1977.
Anticoagulant activity of heparin: assay of bovine, human and porcine preparations by amidolytic and clotting methods.
A: 1.3, 2.3, S: 1, 11.
Teien AN, Abildgaard U, Ødegard OR, Lie M: In I Witt (ed). New Methods for the Analysis of Coagulation using Chromogenic Substrates. de Gruyter, Berlin, 1977, pp 221–227.
Heparin assay in plasma.
A: 2.3, S: 1.
Teien AN, Lie M: Thromb Res 10:399–410, 1977.
Evaluation of an amidolytic heparin assay method: increased sensitivity by adding purified antithrombin III.
A: 2.3, S: 1.

164

Teien AN, Lie M, Abildgaard U: Thromb Res 8:413–416, 1976.
Assay of heparin in plasma using a chromogenic substrate for activated factor X.
A: 2.3, S: 1.

Ten Cate JW: *In* HR Lijnen, D Collen, M Verstraete (eds). Synthetic Substrates in Clinical Blood Coagulation Assays. Martinus Nijhoff Publishers, The Hague, 1980, pp 44–50.
An automated chromogenic antithrombin III method: clinical experience.
A: 1.3, S: 8.

Ten Cate JW, Kahlé LH, Büller HR, Peters M, Weenink GH: Thrombos Haemostas 46:327, 1981 (Meeting abstract).
Clinical information from screening programs for coagulation and fibrinolytic factors and inhibitor deficiences using automated chromogenic methods.
A: 7.

Thomas LLM, Buller HR, Sturk A, ten Cate JW: Brit J Haem 50:689, 1982 (Meeting abstract).
Quantitative endotoxin determination in blood with a chromogenic substrate, relation with antithrombin III (AT-III), plasminogen (PLG) and septicemia.
A: 5.3, S: 1.

Thomas LLM, Sturk A, Schaap MC, Ten Cate H, Ten Cate JW: Thrombos Haemostas 46:314, 1981 (Meeting abstract).
Quantitative endotoxin determination in blood with a chromogenic substrate.
A: 5.3, S: 1.

Triplett DA, Harms C: Thrombos Haemostas 42:20, 1979 (Meeting abstract).
Clinical studies of the use of a fluorogenic substrate assay for the determination of antithrombin III activity.
A: 1.3, S: 16.

Triplett DA, Harms C: Thrombos Haemostas 42:308, 1979 (Meeting abstract).
The use of the fluorogenic synthetic substrate assay for the clinical determination of heparin.
A: 1.3, S: 16.

Triplett DA, Harms C, Hermelin L: Thrombos Haemostas 42:50, 1979 (Meeting abstract).
Clinical studies of the use of a fluorogenic substrate assay method for the determination of plasminogen.
A: 3.2, S: 16.

Triplett DA, Smith C, Harms CS: Am J Clin Pathol 71:613, 1979.
Assay for prothrombin utilizing synthetic substrate S 2238.
A: 1.2, S: 8.

Tripodi A, Di Santo C, Mannucci PM: Ric CL Lab 11:215–222, 1981.
A chromogenic assay of prothrombin compared with coagulation tests during anticoagulant therapy and liver disease.
A: 1.2, S: 9.

Trobisch H, Klasing KH, Richter O: Blut 40:38, 1980 (Meeting abstract).
Zum Mechanismus des Inaktivierung des Faktors X_a durch das progressive Antithrombin (AT III) und den AT III: Heparin Komplex.
A: 2.3, S: 1.

Ts'ao C, Galluzzo TS: Am J Clin Pathol 75:372–377, 1981.
H-D-val-leu-lys-aminoisophtalic acid-dimethyl ester, is sensitive to streptokinase-activator not to plasmin.
A: 3.4, S: 16.

Uchida Y, Oh-Ishi S, Tanaka K, Harada Y, Ueno A, Katori M, Funahashi S, Hashimoto T, Ueno T, Kodama J: *In* S Fujii, H Moriya, T Suzuki (eds). Kinins-II, Biochemistry, Pathophysiology and Clinical Aspects. Plenum Press, New York, 1979, pp 173–184.

Assay methods for prekallikrein and kininogens and their applications.
A: 4.1, S: 16.
Uchida Y, Oh-Ishi S, Tanaka K, Harada Y, Ueno A, Katori M, Funahashi S, Hashimoto T, Ueno T, Kodama J: Adv Exp Med Biol 120A:173–184, 1980.
Assay methods for prekallikrein and kininogens and their applications.
A: 4.1, S: 16.
Uhlmeyer KA, Edlefson DS, Aiyappa PA: Am J Med TE 47:655, 1981 (Meeting abstract).
Evaluation of contact activation in evacuated tubes by a chromogenic substrate assay equivalent to the non-activated partial thromboplastin time.
A: 8.
Umlass J, Gauvin G, Taff R: Am J Clin P 78:271, 1982 (Meeting abstract).
Rapid heparin monitoring and neutralization during cardiopulmonary bypass using rapid plasma separator and a fluorometric heparin assay.
A: 1.3, S: 16.

Vinazzer H, Thromb Diath Haemorrh 34:344, 1975 (Meeting abstract).
Photometric assay of Antithrombin III with a chromogenic substrate.
A: 1.3, S: 11.
Vinazzer H: Haemostasis 4:101–109, 1975.
Photometric assay of antithrombin III with a chromogenic substrate.
A: 1.3, S: 11.
Vinazzer H: Haemostasis 6:283–293, 1977.
Photometric assay of platelet factor 4 with a chromogenic substrate.
A: 2.3, S: 1.
Vinazzer H: In I Witt (ed). New Methods for the Analysis of Coagulation using Chromogenic Substrates. de Gruyter, Berlin, 1977, pp 203–209.
Assay of factor X_a with a chromogenic substrate.
A: 2.1, S: 1.
Vinazzer H: In I Witt (ed). New Methods for the Analysis of Coagulation using Chromogen Substrates. de Gruyter, Berlin, 1977, pp 61–68.
Assay of antithrombin III with the chromogenic substrate S 2160.
A: 1.3, S: 11.
Vinazzer H: Haemostasis 7:352–358, 1978.
A simplified assay method for platelet factor 4 in plasma and in platelets with a chromogenic substrate.
A: 2.3, S: 1.
Vinazzer H: Thrombos Haemostas 42:238, 1979 (Meeting abstract).
Photometric assay of factor VIIIC with a chromogenic substrate.
A: 2.6, S: 1.
Vinazzer H: Thromb Res 14:155–166, 1979.
Assay of total factor XII and of activated factor XII in plasma with a chromogenic substrate.
A: 4.2, S: 7.
Vinazzer H: Haematologica (Pavia) 65:636–643, 1981.
Diagnosis of intravascula coagulation by assays of activated factors X and XII with chromogenic substrates.
A: 2.1, 4.2, S: 1, 7.
Vinazzer H, Heimburger N: Thromb Res 12:503–510, 1978.
Assay of factor X_a in intact plasma as a possible method for early diagnosis of intravascular coagulation.
A: 2.1, S: 1.
Vliet HHDM van: In HR Lijnen, D Collen M Verstraete (eds). Synthetic Substrates in Clinical Blood Coagulation Assays. Martinus Nijhoff Publishers, The Hague, 1980, pp 103–112.

Experience with the determination of kallikrein, plasminogen and antiplasmin using chromogenic substrates: clinical application.
A: 3.1, 3.2, 3.3, 4.1, S: 6, 7, 12, 13.

Walenga J, Fareed J, Messmore HL, Kniffin J: Thrombos Haemostas 46:362, 1981 (Meeting abstract).
Synthetic peptide assays for monitoring the defects of extrinsic and intrinsic pathways of coagulation: selection of a suitable substrate.
A: 7, S: 10, 19.

Walenga J, Fareed J, Messmore HL, Kniffin J, Bermes EW: Clin Chem 27:1107, 1981 (Meeting abstract).
Inhibition of activated factor X_a by thrombin specific synthetic peptide-substrates-implications on the development of global tests for coagulation assays.
A: 7.

Walenga J, Fareed J, Messmore HL, Kniffin J: J Clin Chem Clin Biochem 19:868, 1981 (Meeting abstract).
Chromogenic peptide assays for testing the alterations of extrinsic and intrinsic pathways of coagulation. Selection of a suitable substrate.
A: 7, 8, S: 8, 9, 10, 11, 19.

Walenga J, Fareed J, Messmore HL, Statland BE, Solomon J, Ito R, Perry JF, Wehrly JA: J Clin Chem Clin Biochem 19:868—869, 1981 (Meeting abstract).
An automated Antithrombin III Assay: Analytical Performance and Initial Clinical Studies.
A: 9.

Walz DA, Seegers WH, Reuterby J, McCoy LE: Thromb Res 4:713—717, 1974.
A: 9.

Weinand HA, Haberland K: Blut 40:68, 1980 (Meeting abstract).
Die Bestimmung von Antithrombin III und Heparin mit chromogenen Substraten vor und während der Dialyse.
A: 7.

Weinstein MJ, Doolittle RF: Biochim Biophys Acta 258:577, 1972.
Differential specificities of thrombin, plasmin and trypsin with regard to synthetic and natural substrates and inhibitors.
A: 7.

Wenzel E, Pfordt L, Wenig Ch, Nienhaus KH: *In* I Witt (ed). New Methods for the Analysis of Coagulation using Chromogenic Substrates. de Gruyter, Berlin, 1977, pp 69—89.
Effects of thrombin and low heparin concentrations on the antithrombin activity in human plasma.
A: 1.3, S: 9.

Wenzel E, Svendsen L, Nienhaus KH, Pfordt L: Thrombos Haemostas 38:21, 1977 (Meeting abstract).
Photometric measurement of urokinase and similar activities with a new artificial chromogenic substrate.
A: 3.4, S: 4.

Whur P, Magudia M, Boston J, Lockwood J, Williams DC: Br J Cancer 42:305—313, 1981.
Plasminogen activator in cultured Lewis lung carcinoma cells measured by chromogenic substrate assay.
A: 3.4, S: 12.

Wiman B, Collen D: Eur J Biochem 84:573—578, 1978.
On the kinetics of the reaction between human antiplasmin and plasmin.
A: 7, S: 12.

Witt I: Aktuelle Diagnostik, Boehringer Mannheim, 1976.
Biochemische Grundlagen der Gerinnungsdiagnostik mit chromogene Substraten.
A: 7.

Witt I: *In* I Witt (ed). New Methods for the Analysis of Coagulation using Chromogenic Substrates. de Gruyter, Berlin, 1977, pp 155–169.
Determination of plasma prothrombin with chromozym TH.
A: 1.2, S: 9.

Witt I, Svendsen L: Aktuelle Diagnostick, Boehringer Mannheim, 1977.
Plasma Kallikrein.
A: 4.1, S: 6.

Witt I, Lill H, Karitzky D, Flad H: Thrombos Haemostas 42:124, 1979 (Meeting abstract).
Determination of α-antitrypsin with a chromogenic peptide substrate: methodology and clinical application.
A: 6, S: 19.

Witte DL, Noorbakh M, Owen WG: Clin Chem 25:1147, 1979 (Meeting abstract).
Measurement of antithrombin III by esterolytic, chromogenic and coagulation methodologies.
A: 1.3.

Wohl RC, Arzadon L, Summaria L, Robbins KC: J Biol Chem 252:1141–1147, 1979.
Comparison of the esterase and human plasminogen activator activities of various activated forms of human plasminogen and their equimolar streptokinase complexes.
A: 7, S: 17.

Wohl RC, Summaria L, Arzadon L, Robbins KC: J Biol Chem 253:1402–1407, 1978.
Steady state kinetics of activation of human and bovine plasminogens by forms of human plasminogen.
A: 7, S: 17.

Wohl RC, Summaria L, Robbins KC: J Biol Chem 255:2005–2013, 1980.
Kinetics of activation of human plasminogen by different activator species at pH 7.4 and 37°C.
A: 7, S: 3, 12, 13.

Wijk EM, Kahlé LH, Ten Cate JW: Thrombos Haemostas 42:55, 1979 (Meeting abstract).
The determination of factor X using an automated amidolytic technique.
A: 2.2, S: 1.

Wijk EM van, Kahlé LH, Ten Cate JW: Clin Chem 26:885–890, 1980.
Mechanized amidolytic technique for determination of factor X and factor-X antigen, and its application to patients being treated with oral anticoagulants.
A: 2.2, S: 1.

Wijk EM van, Kahlé LH, Ten Cate JW: Thromb Res 22:681–686, 1981.
A rapid manual chromogenic factor X assay. (Brief communication).
A: 2.2, S: 2.

Wijk EM van, Kahlé LH, Jeletich A, Ten Cate JW: Thrombos Haemostas 46:364, 1981 (Meeting abstract).
A comparison between thrombotest and factor-X amidolytic activity in stable and non-stable anticoagulated patients.
A: 2.2.

Wijk EM van, Kahlé LH, Jeletich A, Ten Cate JW: Sc J Haemat 29:105–114, 1982.
Further evaluation of an automated amidolytic factor-X assay in monitoring anti-vitamin-K treatment.
A: 2.2, S: 2.

Wijk EM van, Kahlé LH, Wiebosch M, Ten Cate JW: Clin Chem 27:918–921, 1981.
Optimization of a mechanized amidolytic factor-X assay-influence of reaction conditions and reagents.
A: 2.2, S: 1.

Wijngaards G, Nieuwenhuizen W: *In* HR Lijnen, D Collen, M Verstraete (eds). Synthetic Substrates in Clinical Blood Coagulation Assays. Martinus Nijhoff Publishers, The Hague, 1980, pp 123–131.
Fluorogenic substrates and the assay of urokinase and tissue plasminogen activator.
A: 3.4, S: 16.

Yamada K, Meguro T: Thrombos Haemostas 42:225, 1979 (Meeting abstract).
Noval method of APTT using the chromogenic substrates for thrombin and an autoanalyzer.
A: 8, S: 8.
Yamada K, Meguro T: Thromb Res 15:351–358, 1979.
A new APTT assay employing a chromogenic substrate and a centrifugal autoanalyzer.
A: 8, S: 8.
Yamamoto T, Kozono K, Okamoto T, Kato H, Kambara T: Biochim Biophys Acta 614:511–525, 1981.
Purification of guinea-pig plasma prekallikrein. Activation by prekallikrein activator derived from guinea-pig skin.
A: 4.1, S: 16.
Yoshida N: Acta Haem Jap 40:197, 1977.
Effects of α_2-macroglobulin and FDP on the antithrombin III assay-system.
A: 9.
Yue RH, Gertler MM: J Am Med A 242:1360–1361, 1979.
Antithrombin-III assays.
A: 7.

Zimmerman M, Ashe B, Yurewicz EC, Patel G: Anal Biochem 78:47–51, 1977.
Sensitive assays for trypsin, elastase and chymotrypsin using new fluorogenic substrates.
A: 6, S: 16.
Zimmerman RE, Schwering H, Wittrin G, Hollenders Th: Chirurg 52:316–319, 1981.
(GE) Control of low-dose heparin-therapy by photometric detection of biologically active heparin.
A: 2.3, S: 1.
Zimmerman M, Yurewicz EC, Patel C: Anal Biochem 70:258–262, 1976.
A new fluorogenic substrate for chymotrypsin.
A: 6, S: 16.
Zimmerman M, Quigley JP, Ashe B, Dorn C, Goldfarb R, Troll W: Proc Natl Acad Sci USA 75:750–753, 1978.
Direct fluorescent assay of urokinase and plasminogen activators of normal and malignant cells: kinetics and inhibitor profiles.
A: 3.4, S: 16.
Zuffi T, Jordan R: Thrombos Haemostas 46:231, 1981 (Meeting abstract).
Direct assay for factor XII in plasma.
A: 4.2, S: 7.
Zur M, Nemerson Y: J Biol Chem 253:2203–2209, 1978.
The esterase activity of coagulation factor VII. Evidence for intrinsic activity of the zymogen.
A: 7.

INDEX OF SUBJECTS

absolute temperature, 34

absorbance, 28, 30

absorbance range, 32

absorbency index, 29

absorbency maximum, 33

absorption, 27

absorption maximum, 27

absorption spectrophotometry, 28

absorption spectrum, 27, 28

accessory binding site, 54

α_1-acid glycoprotein, 107

acid hydrolysis of the substrate, 37

activated partial thromboplastin time, 106

active centre, 12

active enzyme molecules, 19

active serine, 53, 54

active site, 3, 21, 54

active site titrants, 21, 22, 59

active site titration, 19

acylenzyme intermediate, 13

Affi-gel: AGIO, 91

AGIO-Ala-Ala-Ala-Phe-IL, 91

AGIO-Ala-Phe-Pro-Arg-IL, 91

AIE 5 amino isophtalic acid dimethyl ester, 86

aldrithiol-4, 88

amide substrate, 15, 17

aminoisophtalic acid, 83

amino acid thioester substrate, 89

ϵ-amino caproic acid, 59

7-amino-4-methylcoumarin (AMC), 83, 84, 85

5-amino-isophtalic acid dimethylester (AIE), 83, 84

amino-peptidase, 83

7-amino-4-trifluorocarbon coumarine (TFCA), 84

amplification of colour yield after the splitting of chromogenic substrates, 126

anti-antithrombin III immunoglobulin, 103

α_1-antichymotrypsin, 120

Antifactor X_a (antithrombin III, heparin cofactor), 104

antiheparins, 106, 125

anti Pf 4 antibody, 107

antiplasmin, 125

α_2-antiplasmin, 120

antithrombin III, 50, 98, 99, 103, 105, 107, 120, 121, 125

α_1-antitrypsin, 120

aprotinin, 36, 59

APTT, 106

Arrhenius plot, 34

Arvin, 98

Aspergillus oryzae, 118

bacterial endotoxin, 119, 125

BAM, 15

bandwidth, 32

Batter's syndrome, 118

Basic enzymology, 1

bentonite, 98

b-Ile-Glu(pip)-Glu-Arg-pNA.HCl, 69

b-Ile-Glu-Gly-Arg-pNA.HCl, 66, 67

b-Ile-Pip-Gly-Arg-pNA, 66

billirubin, 106

boar acrosin, 22

Boc-Ala-Ala-Phe-IL, 91

Boc-Glu-Lys-Lys-MCA, 88

Boc-Glu-(OBz)-Gly-Arg-MCA, 115, 116

Boc-Ile-Glu-Gly-Arg-MCA, 87

Boc-Leu-Gly-Arg-MCA, 87, 119, 120

Boc-Leu-Ser-Thr-Arg-MCA, 88

Boc-Leu-Thr-Arg-MCA, 88
Boc-Phe-Glu-Lys-Lys-MCA, 88
Boc-Phe-Ser-Arg-MCA, 88, 116, 117
Boc-Ser-Gly-Arg-MCA, 87
Boc-Val-Gly-Arg-βNA, 86
Boc-Val-Leu-Lys-MCA, 88
Boc-Val-Pro-Arg-MCA, 87
bovine pancreatic trypsin inhibitor, 118
b-Phe-Leu-Arg-pNA, 78
b-Phe-Val-Arg-pNA, 66
b-Pro-Phe-Arg-pNA, 66
b-Pro-Phe-Arg-pNA.HCl, 73
brinase, 36, 118, 125
brinase inhibitors, 118, 125
b-Val-Gly-Arg-pNA.HCl, 66, 71
Bz-Ile-Glu(pip)-Gly-Arg-pADA.2HCl, 89

calibration curve, 50
carbobenzoxy (Z)-Phe-Arg-MCA, 113
carbowax 6000, 36, 96
casein, 56
catalytic activity, 18
catalytic mechanism, 53
catalytic rate constant, 12
cathepsin G, 81
Cbz-Ala-Ala-Lys-MβNA, 86
Cbz-Gly-Gly-Arg-MCA, 87
Cbz-Gly-Gly-Arg-TFCA, 86
Cbz-Gly-Pro-Arg-βNA, 86
Cbz-Gly-Pro-Arg(HCC)-4 methody B
    naphtylamide, 99
Cbz-Phe-Arg-MCA, 87
Cbz-Pro-Phe-Arg-MCA, 87
celite eluate, 113
Cephotest (Nygaard), 113
1-chloro-3-tosylamido-7-aminoheptane
    (TLCK), 22
choice of wavelength, 32
chromogenic substrate, 13, 14, 15,
    17, 21, 23, 24, 32, 34, 38, 53,
    56, 59, 95, 119
chromokallikrein, 73
chromoplasmin, 80
chromothrombin, 76
chromozym PK, 66, 113, 115, 126
chromozym PL, 66, 73, 80, 126
chromozym TH, 27, 28, 29, 62, 66,
    75, 76, 99, 126
chromozym Try, 71
chromozym UK, 66, 71, 119, 126

chymotrypsin, 22, 55, 66, 81, 82,
    83, 88, 91
clotting enzyme, 125
clotting enzyme in the hemocyte lysate
    from the horseshoe crab, 119
cmprop-Arg-Pro-Tyr-pNA.HCl, 66, 81
coagulase-thrombin, 95
coagulation enzymes, 42, 54
coagulation proteases, 55
coagulation reaction, 34
Coatest® /heparin Kabivitrium, 106
Coatest Kabivitrium®, 105
collagen, 107
collagen suspension, 101
collision frequencies, 3
commercially available substrates, 65
commercial filters, 33
competitive inhibition, 10
competitive inhibitor, 23, 63
competitive reversible inhibitors, 59
contact activation system, 112
contact phase of blood coagulation, 115
contaminating enzyme, 24
conversion of a chromogenic
    substrate, 27
coumarin derivatives, 83
covalent tetrahedral complex, 13
criteria of homogeneity, 18
CTA, 112
C 1s, 77
C 2s, 77
C$_1$-inhibitor, 120

decarboxy factor X (PIVKA-X), 103
decarboxy-prothrombin, 96, 97
destruction by light, 37
difference spectrum, 31, 32
diisopropylfluorophosphate (DFP), 22, 59
D-Ile-Pro-Arg-pNA.HCl, 66, 77
dimethylformamide, 116
dimethylsulfoxide, 113
dipeptide thioester substrates, 89
Dl.BAPADA, 89
4,4'-dithiopyridine (Aldrithiol-4), 88, 89
D.L. Benzoylarginine HCl, 89
DMSO, 89, 91
D-Phe-Pip-Arg-pNA, 66
D-Pro-Phe-Arg-pNA, 66
dual wavelength measurements, 31, 32
D-Val-Gly-Arg-pNA, 66

D-Val-Leu-Lys-pNA.2HCl, 66, 79

Ecarin (Echis carinatus venom), 96, 97
efficiency constant, 5, 23, 89
efficiency of the enzym, 5, 6, 16
elastase, 55, 81, 83, 88
electroanalysis, 47
electrochemical determinations, 47, 48
electrochemical oxidation, 47
electrochemical signal, 50
electrostatic interaction, 56
ellagic acid, 112
emission, 44
endotoxin, 119, 120, 121
endotoxin induced amindase activity, 119
endotoxin sensitive clotting enzyme, 119
endpoint methods, 39, 41, 85
enzyme, 1
enzyme inhibition, 9
enzyme inhibitor complex, 10
enzyme product complex, 2, 4
enzyme substrate complex (ES), 2, 3, 11
epinephrin, 107
epsilonaminocaproic acid (EACA), 113, 115
ethyl-P-guanidinobenzoate, 22
excitation spectrum, 45
execution of the experiment, 38
extinction, 29, 30
extinction coefficient, 29
extrinsic activator, 107

Factor II, 120
Factor II$_a$, 74, 88, 120
Factor V, 97, 99, 100, 101, 120, 125
Factor V$_a$, 120
Factor VII, 97, 103, 109
Factor VII$_a$, 107
Factor VIII, 108, 120, 125
Factor VIII$_a$, 107
Factor IX, 108, 120, 125
Factor IX$_a$, 57, 88, 89, 107, 120, 125
Factor X, 103, 108, 109, 120, 125
Factor X$_a$, 20, 22, 36, 57, 59, 62, 63, 66, 67, 68, 69, 74, 75, 76, 77, 78, 79, 80, 81, 82, 85, 87, 88, 89, 99, 100, 102, 103, 104, 105, 107, 109, 113, 120, 125
Factor XI, 112, 116, 120, 125
Factor XI$_a$, 88, 89, 108, 116, 117, 125

Factor XII, 112, 113, 114, 115, 116, 120, 125
Factor XII$_a$, 74, 77, 88, 89, 114, 115, 116, 117, 120, 125
Factor XIII, 120
Factor XIII*, 120
Factor XIII$_a$, 120
Factor X activating complex, 107, 125
Factor X$_1$, 102
Factor X$_2$, 102
fibrinogen, 55, 97, 120
fibrinolytic pathway components in plasma, 109
filter monochromators, 31
Fitzgerald trait, 112
Fleaujac, 112
Fletcher deficiency, 112
Fletcher factor, 112
Fletcher trait, 114
fluoresceine, 47
fluorescence, 44, 45, 46
fluorescence spectra of peptide MCA and AMC, 85
fluorescence spectrum, 45
fluorimetry, 83
fluorogenic leaving groups, 83
fluorogenic peptide substrates with 7-amino-4-methyl-coumarine as a leaving group, 83
fluorogenic substrate, 59, 83, 118, 119, 126
fluorometric assays, 83
fruitful collision, 2, 12

glandular kallikrein, 66, 72, 117, 120, 125
Glu-Gly-Arg-MCA, 87
Glu-plasminogen, 110
Glu-plasminogen SK, 79, 80
Gly-Arg-βNA, 86
granulocyte elastase, 66, 81, 82
graphic registration, 39

Hageman deficiency, 112
Hageman factor, 87, 114
heating by the incident light beam, 46
hematin, 90, 91
heparin, 99, 104, 105, 106, 107, 125
heparin cofactor, 98, 125
heparin inhibition, 97

high molecular weight kallikrein, 120
high molecular weight kininogen
  (HMWK), 112, 113, 114, 115
hirudin, 36
hog pancreatic kallikrein, 114
horseshoe crab, 125
horseshoe crab clotting enzyme, 85
human salivary kallikrein, 72
hydrolic model, 15
2-hydroxy-p-nitro-α-toluenesulfonic
  acid sulfone, 22
H-binding, 56
H-D-Ala-Leu-Lys-TFCA, 86
H-D-Phe-Pip-Arg-4MeO-napthylamine,
  90
H-D-Phe-Pip-Arg-pADA.2HCl, 89
H-D-Phe-Pip-Arg-pNA.2HCl, 75, 95
H-D-Phe-Pro-Arg-AIA, 86
H-D-Pro-Phe-Arg-pADA, 89
H-D-Pro-Phe-Arg-pNA.2HCl, 74
H-D-Val-Leu-Arg-pADA, 89
H-D-Val-Leu-Arg-pNA.2HCl, 72
H-D-Val-Leu-Lys-AIA, 86
H-D-Val-Leu-Lys-pNA, 110, 111
H-D-Val-Leu-Lys-TFCA, 86
H-TAME, 114
H-Val-Gly-Arg-βNA, 86

infinite substrate concentration, 3
inhibition, 59
inhibition by artificial substrates, 64
inhibitors, 9, 36, 125
initial burst, 15, 19
initial phase of the reaction, 14
initial rate method, 85, 116
initial reaction rate, 7, 11
initial reaction velocity, 37, 42, 60
intensity, 29
interface current, 48
international unit of enzyme activity, 42
interval measurement, 39
inter-α-trypsin inhibitor, 120
intrinsic activator, 107
inverse form of the Michaelis-Menten
  relationship, 8
ionic strength, 35, 37
IOWA-unit, 97
irreversible inhibitor, 10, 15, 58
isoluminolamide (IL), 90
isosbestic point, 30, 31, 32

Kabivitrium Coatest®/Factor X, 104
kallikrein, 36, 57, 79, 81, 82, 85,
  114, 115, 116, 117, 118
kallikrein inhibitors, 125
Kallikrein Pl, 89
Kallikrein U, 89
Kaolin, 113, 114, 115
katal, 42
k_{cat}, 4, 8, 10, 12, 15, 21, 23, 24,
  35, 42, 58, 61, 62, 65
kinetic analysis, 59
kinetic constants, 18, 33, 37, 65, 89
kinetic parameters, 18, 59, 60
K_m, 5, 8, 10, 15, 16, 18, 23, 24,
  25, 35, 36, 42, 61, 62, 63, 65

lag phases, 41
Lambert-Beer's law, 28, 32
leaving group, 54
Lee and Wilson type of evaluation of
  experimental data, 42
length measurement, 32
level of specificity, 55
lifetime of the enzyme-substrate complex, 3
light intensity, 31
lima bean trypsin inhibitor (LBTI),
  59, 113, 114
Limulus enzyme, 87
limulus hemocyte lysate, 119
Limulus polyphemus, 119
Limulus test, 121
linear part of the reaction, 36
Lineweaver-Burk plot, 8, 10, 25
liver disease, 96
low molecular weight kallikrein, 120
luminescent leaving group, 90
luminogenic assay, 90
luminogenic substrates, 90, 91, 126
Lys-Plasmin SK, 79

α_2-macroglobulin, 103, 104, 120
mathematical procedures, 8
maximal velocity, 3
MCA (7-amino-4-methylcoumarine), 87
mean concentration, 37
mean velocity, 37
mean velocity over a certain time lapse, 37
meizothrombin, 95
MeOSuc-Ala-Phe-Lys-MCA, 88
4-methoxy-2-naphtylamine, 84

4-methyl-2-naphtylamine (MβNA), 86
4-methylumbelliferyl-p-ω-dimethyl-
    sulfonioacetamidobenzoate, 22
methylumbelliferyl-p-guanidino-
    benzoate, 22
4-methylumbelliferyl-(N,N,N-triethyl-
    amonium)cinnamate, 22
Michaelis complex, 13
Michaelis-Menten kinetics, 8
Michaelis-Menten relationship, 5, 7,
    8, 37, 42, 60
microbial growth, 38
α_2M inhibitor-brinase complex, 119
molar absorbence index, 29
molar absorbtivity, 29, 30, 31
molar absorption, 32
molar extinction, 31
molecular extinction coefficient, 29, 47
monochromatic light, 32
mutual competitive inhibition, 65

Na-azide, 36
naphtylamines, 83, 84
natural substrate, 24
N-benzyloxycarbonyl-L-tyrosine-p-
    nitrophenylester, 22
N-benz-NO$_2$Phe-Val-Arg-pNA.HCl
    (S2160), 95
Nα-Cbz-L-lysine-p-nitrophenylester, 110
NIH units, 97
Nα-methyl-Nα-toluenesulfonyl-L-lysine-
    α-naphtylester, 22
noncovalent bonds, 12
noncovalent enzyme-substrate complex
    (Michaelis complex), 12, 13
nonspecific absorption, 31
non-competitive inhibitor, 10
non-competitive reversible inhibitors, 59
non-enzymatic acid hydrolysis of the
    substrate, 39
N-tos-Gly-Pro-Arg-pNA.HCl
    (chromozym TH), 95
nucleophilicity, 54

opalescent solution, 45
optical density, 29
oral anticoagulation, 96
ovalbumin, 36, 96, 101, 102, 108

pADA, 47, 50, 89

p-aminodiphenylamine (pADA), 47, 50,
    89
pancreas elastase, 82
pancreatic basic trypsin inhibitor
    (Trasylol®), 116
pancreatic kallikrein, 87
pancreatic kallikrein(hog), 87
papain, 36
peptide argininaldehydes, 58
peptide chloromethylketones, 58
peptidylarginine chloromethylketones, 59
Pf 4, 107
pGlu-Gly-Arg-pNA.HCl, 66, 70
pGlu-Pro-Val-pNA, 66, 82
phospholipid, 99, 100, 107
phospholipid suspension, 101, 108
photometric assay, 27
pH, 35, 37
pharmacological bioassay, 44
PIVKA, 96
plasma, 116
plasma kallikrein, 22, 66, 68, 73, 74,
    77, 87, 88, 112, 125
plasma prekallikrein, 112, 113, 125
plasmin, 22, 35, 36, 55, 56, 58, 59,
    68, 73, 74, 76, 77, 78, 79, 80, 81,
    82, 85, 86, 87, 88, 89, 111, 112,
    113, 114, 115, 120, 125
α_2-plasmin inhibitor, 111, 112, 121
plasmin B chain SK, 79
plasmin generation, 111
plasminogen, 109, 110, 111, 112, 120
plasminogen activators, 110, 125
Plasmogen SK, 79
platelet factor 3, 99, 100, 101, 108, 125
platelet factor 4 (Pf 4), 106
platelet prothrombin convertin activity,
    102
Ploug U., 112
p-nitroaniline, 13, 27, 28, 32, 39
p-nitrophenyl ethyl diazomalonate, 22
p-nitrophenyl-N-acetyl-DL-trypto-
    phanate, 22
p-nitrophenyl-N^2-acetyl-N^1-benzylcar-
    bazate, 22
p-nitrophenyl-Nα-benzyloxycarbonyl-
    L-lysinate HCl, 22
p-nitrophenyl-N-benzyloxycarbonyl-
    L-tyrosinate, 22
p-nitrophenyl-p^1-amidinobenzoate HCl, 22

p-nitrophenyl-p-guanidinobenzoate HCl (p-NPGB), 21, 22
p-nitrophenyl trimethylacetate, 22
polybrene, 97, 99, 104
polyethyleneglycol PEG), 36
polypeptide inhibitors, 15
potential difference, 47
Pregel®, 120
prekallikrein, 89, 114, 115, 120
presteady state, 17
primary structure, 18, 56
prism monochromators, 31
productive enzyme substrate complex, 5
product inhibition, 42
progress curve, 60
prostaglandin E, 106
protein C, 88
proteolytic enzymes, 2, 83
proteolytic inhibitors, 18
prothrombin, 96, 97, 98, 125
prothrombinase complex, 24, 43, 58, 97, 99, 100, 125
Pro-Phe-Arg-MCA, 87, 117, 118
pseudo-substrates, 59
pyroglutamyl peptidase, 83

quantum efficiency of fluorescence, 47
quantum yield, 46, 47
quinine, 47

Raman effect, 45
Raman scattering, 44
Rayleigh scattering, 44, 45
reaction medium, 35, 38, 46
reaction velocity, 21, 34
release reaction of platelets, 106
reversible inhibitors, 59
Russell's Viper Venom (RVV, Stypven), 97, 99, 101, 103

saturation curve, 6
scattering in the sample, 31, 32, 45
second level of specificity, 55
selectivity, 53, 57, 58
sensitivity, 31, 45, 58
serine protease, 1, 12, 14, 17, 18, 21, 22, 53, 55, 77, 78, 88
serum albumin, 36
simultaneous reactions, 21
small ester substrates, 126

snake venoms, 96
soy bean trypsin inhibitor (SBTI), 15, 56, 59, 96, 113, 114, 117
species specificity, 109
specificity, 45, 53, 57
specificity in serine proteases, 53
specific inhibitors, 58
spectrophotometric measurement, 31
standard plasma, 43
staphylocoagulase, 96
steady phase, 19
steady state conditions, 11
streptokinase, 110, 111, 120
strip chart recording, 40
subsite, 54
substrates, 53
substrates for electrochemical determinations, 89
substrate selectivity and -sensitivity, 57
substrate solution, 36
Succinoyl-Ala-Phe-Lys-MCA, 88
synthetic substrates, 125, 126
S 2160, 66, 78, 99, 118, 126
S 2222, 57, 62, 63, 66, 67, 103, 104, 105, 107, 108, 109, 126
S 2226, 72
S 2237, 102
S 2238, 50, 66, 75, 78, 86, 96, 98, 99, 101, 126
S 2251, 66, 79, 86, 126
S 2266, 66, 117, 126
S 2288, 66, 77, 126
S 2302, 57, 74, 112, 115, 126
S 2303, 66
S 2337, 66, 69, 126
S 2421, 90
S 2444, 57, 66, 70, 126
S 2484, 66, 82, 126
S 2497, 49, 50, 51, 89
S 2586, 66, 81, 126
S 2644, 89
S 2646, 89
S 2648, 89
S 2649, 89

Tachypleus tridentatus, 119
Taipan snake, 96
TAMe, 15
temperature, 33, 45
temperature dependence of protein

denaturation, 35
temperature dependency, 34
tenase complex, 107, 108
tertiary structure, 18, 56
tetrahedral complex, 54
TFCA (7-amino-4-trifluorocarbonyl-
    coumarin), 86
theophylline, 106
thioester, 88
thioester substrates, 126
third level of specificity, 55
t-Gly-Pro-Arg-pNA.HCl, 66, 76
t-Gly-Pro-Lys-pNA.HCl, 66, 80
thrombin, 22, 36, 49, 54, 55, 57, 58,
    62, 63, 66, 68, 69, 75, 76, 77, 78,
    79, 80, 81, 82, 83, 86, 87, 89, 91,
    95, 96, 98, 125
thrombin and derived determinations, 95
thrombin generation, 43, 44
thrombolytic agent, 118
thromboplastin, 97, 103, 107, 108, 109
thrombotest, 97
tissue activator, 86
tissue kallikreins, 117
tissue thromboplastin, 108
tosyl arginine methyl ester (TAMe), 59
TPA-1ch, 77
TPA-2ch, 77
transient phase, 19
transient state, 11, 17
transient state kinetics, 16
trans-cinnamoyl imidazole, 22
transmission, 29
Trasylol®, 59, 111, 118

triangular signal, 48
trypsin, 22, 36, 54, 55, 56, 57, 68,
    70, 73, 74, 76, 78, 79, 80, 81, 86,
    87, 88, 89, 91, 116, 117
turbidity, 31, 32
turbid media, 31
turnover number, 4, 16
two stage assays, 38

ultraviolet spectra of peptide MCA
    and AMC, 85
uncompetitive inhibitor, 10
unfruitful collisions, 4
unfruitful dissociations of the complex, 4
urinary kallikrein, 87, 117
urine, 118
urokinase, 35, 36, 66, 70, 71, 72, 73,
    75, 79, 80, 81, 82, 85, 86, 87, 88,
    110, 111, 117, 118

Val 442-Plasmin SK, 79
Val 443-Plasmogen-SK, 79
vitamin K deficiency, 96
V_{max}, 4, 8, 18, 25, 42

v.d. Waals interaction, 56
Williams traint, 112
WHO unit, 97

X-propyl dipeptidase, 83

Z-Ala-Ala-Phe-IL, 91
Z-Phe-Arg-MCA, 114
Z-Phe-Pro-Arg-IL, 91